Linda Spencer, LAc
570-724-7817
Wellsboro & Williamsport, Pa

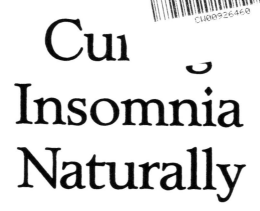

Cur Insomnia Naturally

with
Chinese Medicine

Bob Flaws

BLUE POPPY PRESS

Published by:

BLUE POPPY PRESS
A Division of Blue Poppy Enterprises, Inc.
5441 Western Ave., #2
BOULDER, CO 80301

First Edition, November, 1997
Second Printing, March 2005
Third Printing, February 2006
Fourth Printing, November 2007

ISBN 0-936185-86-4
ISBN 978-0-936185-86-6
LC# 97-71729

Warning: When following some of the self-care techniques given in this book, failure to follow the author's instruction may result in side effects or negative reactions. Therefore, please be sure to follow the author's instructioncarefully for all self-care techniques and modalities. For instance, wrong or excessive application of moxibustion may cause local burns with redness, inflammation, blistering, or even possible scarring. If you have any questions about doing these techniques safely and without unwanted side effects, please see a local professional practitioner for instruction.

Disclaimer: The information in this book is given in good faith. However, the translators and the publishers cannot be held responsible for any error or omission. Nor can they be held in any way responsible for treatment given on the basis of information contained in this book. The publishers make this information available to English language readers for scholarly and research purposes only.

COMP Designation: Original work using a standard translational terminology

Cover design by Eric Brearton

Printed at National Hirschfeld, LLC, Denver, CO

10 9 8 7 6 5 4

Other books in this series include:
Curing Arthritis Fever Naturally with Chinese Medicine
Curing Hay Fever Naturally with Chinese Medicine
Curing Headaches Naturally with Chinese Medicine
Better Breast Health Naturally with Chinese Medicine
Curing Depression Naturally with Chinese Medicine
Curing IBS Naturally with Chinese Medicine
Curing PMS Naturally with Chinese Medicine
Managing Menopause Naturally with Chinese Medicine
Curing Fibromyalgia Naturally with Chinese Medicine
Controlling Diabetes Naturally with Chinese Medicine

Preface

I have been practicing traditional Chinese medicine in the United States of America for almost 20 years. During that time, I have mostly specialized in Chinese medical gynecology, pediatrics, and what Chinese doctors call internal medicine. Insomnia, called either *bu mian*, no sleep, or *shi mian*, loss of sleep in Chinese, has been one of Chinese medicine's core internal diseases for not less than 2,000 years.

Although I have written numerous textbooks and clinical manuals for professionals on all aspects of Chinese medicine, up till now, there has not been any simple discussion of the Chinese medical diagnosis and treatment of insomnia written specifically for the lay reader. Therefore, I have created this book for sufferers of insomnia, their friends, and families. Hopefully, the reader will find that traditional Chinese medicine is an enlightening and empowering alternative or complement to more conventional treatment. Chinese medicine has a whole and holistic, centuries old, well developed and coherent theory about the cause and treatment of insomnia. Not only is this theory enlightening, providing as it does an entirely different perspective on this common complaint from modern Western medicine, it is also empowering. Based on this theory, the reader will find there are all sorts of things, most of which are free or very low cost, which they can do for themselves in order to relieve and even cure their insomnia.

Insomnia does not have to occur. If it does, Chinese medicine has ways to cure or alleviate it.

Bob Flaws
Boulder, CO
March 1997

Table of Contents

Introduction

Jocelyne was distraught. She had been tossing and turning in bed for hours. The clock by her bedside said it was 3:00 AM, and tomorrow she had to give an important presentation. How was she ever going to be able to pull it off unless she fell asleep immediately? However, the more she fretted over not being able to sleep, the more tense and awake she became. What was worse, Jocelyne hadn't been able to get a good night's sleep in weeks. During the day, she was exhausted, but, when it came time to lay down at night, her mind would not turn off and her eyes would not close. It was getting so that she dreaded the coming of bedtime and the special torture of sleeplessness it brought.

Sound familiar? If so, this book may very well help you break the cycle of insomnia. Traditional Chinese doctors have been treating insomnia safely and effectively for tens of centuries.

This book is a layperson's guide to the diagnosis and treatment of insomnia with Chinese medicine. In it, you will learn what causes insomnia *and what you can do about it*. Hopefully, you will be able to identify yourself and your symptoms in these pages. If you can see yourself in the signs and symptoms I discuss below, I feel confident I will be able to share with you a number of self-help techniques which can minimize your discomfort. I have been a professional practitioner of Chinese medicine for almost 20 years, and I have helped scores of Western patients cure or relieve their insomnia. Chinese medicine cannot cure every disease, but when it comes to insomnia, Chinese medicine is the best alternative I know. When someone calls me and says that insomnia is their major complaint, I know that, if they follow my advice, together we can cure or at least reduce their difficulty getting a good night's sleep.

What is insomnia?

According to *The Merck Manual*, the clinical Bible of Western MDs, insomnia refers to "Difficulty in sleeping, or disturbed sleep patterns leaving the perception of insufficient sleep."[1] Insomnia is a common symptom and may be due to a number of emotional and physical disorders.

Types of insomnia

Western medicine recognizes at least three types of insomnia. The first is called initial insomnia. This refers to difficulty falling asleep after having laid down at night. The person cannot enter sleep at night. This is commonly associated with emotional disturbances, such as anxiety, a phobic state, or depression. The second type of insomnia is called matitudinal insomnia or early morning wakening. The person is able to fall asleep, but then they wake up early in the morning, several hours before it is time to arise. Once awake, they then cannot fall back asleep. This pattern of early waking is a common phenomenon of aging. However, even though it is common, it is nonetheless painful for its sufferers. In some cases, this type of insomnia may also be associated with depression. The third type of insomnia is called inverted sleep rhythm. If older patients with insomnia overuse sedative medications, they may be drowsy in the morning and doze all day. Then, when it comes time to sleep at night, they no longer feel tired. If the dose of sedatives is increased, the patient may feel

---

[1] *The Merck Manual of Diagnosis & Therapy*, Robert Berkow, MD, editor, Merck, Sharp & Dohme Research Laboratories, Rahway, NJ, 1987, p. 1376

restless, clouded, dazed, or confused at night. If they suspend their sedative medication, their insomnia tends to return full force.

Causes of insomnia

Some people just sleep less than others. When insomnia is longstanding with little apparent relationship to immediate physical or psychological occurrences, this is called primary insomnia. If insomnia is due to pain, anxiety, or depression, this is called secondary insomnia. In other words, the insomnia is secondary to some other factor in the person's life. When insomnia is of relatively recent onset, it is usually due to current anxieties, such as marital strife, problems at work, financial troubles, or concern over one's health. However, as we will see below, insomnia may follow a prolonged or extreme febrile (*i.e.*, feverish) disease and may occur in women around the menses, after giving birth, or around or after menopause due to physical events associated with female physiology.

How Western medicine treats insomnia

When Western MDs try to treat insomnia, they usually do so using a combination of nonspecific advice coupled with a prescription for one or more Western pharmaceuticals. By nonspecific advice, I mean generic advice given to all sufferers of insomnia, such as getting more exercise, trying to relax, or drinking warm milk before bed. As we will see below, the Chinese doctor may also give the same advice but on an individualized basis. For some patients, getting more exercise may be good, while for others, it might aggravate their insomnia. Likewise, warm milk may help certain people sleep but worsen others' restlessness at night. Therefore, Chinese doctors give very specific advice to each individual patient.

The Western medications most often prescribed for insomnia are called sedatives and hypnotics. Laypeople often refer to these as tranquilizers. Valium or Diazepam is probably the most often prescribed and best known of these. Unfortunately, all such drugs involve some risk of overdose and addiction. In addition, when discontinued, there are withdrawal symptoms which can include the recurrence of insomnia. Further, because they are sedatives, it is important that persons taking these types of drugs not engage in any activity afterwards which requires mental alertness, judgement, or physical coordination, such as driving.

Some of the common adverse or unwanted side effects of sedatives and hypnotics are drowsiness, lethargy, and "hangover." Less often, there can also be hives, nausea, and vomiting. Ironically, in older patients, any sedative may cause restlessness and overexcitement. It is also sad but true that many patients take higher doses than they should or will admit to, thus causing slurring of speech, lack of coordination, and shaking due to overdose. And finally, sedatives are addicting in the same way that alcohol, opiates, antihistamines, and antidepressants are. Therefore, it is no wonder that many people are afraid or do not want to take sedatives.

Happily, Chinese medicine has a number of safe and effective, low cost and nonaddictive alternatives which have been used in Asia for hundreds and thousands of years.

East is East and West is West

In order for the reader to understand and make sense of the rest of this book on Chinese medicine and insomnia, one must understand that Chinese medicine is a distinct and separate system of medical thought and practice from modern Western medicine. This means that one must shift models of reality when it comes to thinking about Chinese medicine. It has taken the

Chinese more than 2,000 years to develop this medical system. In fact, Chinese medicine is the oldest continually practiced, literate, professional medicine in the world. As such one cannot understand Chinese medicine by trying to explain it in Western scientific or medical terms.

Most people reading this book have probably taken high school biology back when they were sophomores. Whether we recognize it or not, most of us Westerners think of what we learned about the human body in high school as "the really real" description of reality, not one possible description. However, if Chinese medicine is to make any sense to Westerners at all, one must be able to entertain the notion that there are potentially other valid descriptions of the human body, its functions, health, and disease. In grappling with this fundamentally important issue, it is useful to think about the concepts of a map and the terrain it describes.

If we take the United States of America as an example, we can have numerous different maps of this country's land mass. One map might show population. Another might show per capita incomes. Another might show religious or ethnic distributions. Yet another might be a road map. And still another might be a map showing political, *i.e.*, state boundaries. In fact, there could be an infinite number of potentially different maps of the United States depending on what one was trying to show and do. As long as the map is based on accurate information and has been created with self-consistent logic, then one map is not necessarily more correct than another. The issue is to use the right map for what you are trying to do. If one wants to drive from Chicago to Washington, DC, then a road map is probably the right one *for that job* but is not necessarily a truer or "more real" description of the United States than a map showing annual rainfall.

What I am getting at here is that *the map is not the terrain.* The Western biological map of the human body is only one potentially useful medical map. It is no more true than the traditional

Chinese medical map, and the "facts" of one map cannot be reduced to the criteria or standards of another *unless they share the same logic right from the beginning*. As long as the Western medical map is capable of solving a person's disease in a cost-effective, time-efficient manner without side effects or iatrogenesis (meaning doctor-caused disease), then it is a useful map. Chinese medicine needs to be judged in the same way. The Chinese medical map of health and disease is just as "real" as the Western biological map as long as, using it, professional practitioners are able to solve their patients' health problems in a safe and effective way.

Therefore, the following chapter is an introduction to the basics of Chinese medicine. Unless one understands some of the fundamental theories and "facts" of Chinese medicine, one will not be able to understand or accept the reasons for some of the Chinese medical treatments of insomnia. As the reader will quickly see from this brief overview of Chinese medicine, "This doesn't look like Kansas, Toto!"

An Overview of the Chinese Medical Map

In this chapter, we will look at an overview of Chinese medicine. In particular, we will discuss yin and yang, qi, blood, and essence, the viscera and bowels, and the channels and network vessels. In the following chapter, we will go on to see how Chinese medicine views sleep and wakefulness. After that, we will look at the Chinese medical diagnosis and treatment of the various patterns of insomnia identified by professional practitioners of Chinese medicine.

Yin & Yang

To understand Chinese medicine, one must first understand the concepts of yin and yang since these are the most basic concepts in this system. Yin and yang are the cornerstones for understanding, diagnosing, and treating the body and mind in Chinese medicine. In a sense, all the other theories and concepts of Chinese medicine are nothing other than an elaboration of yin and yang. Most people have probably already heard of yin and yang but may have only a fuzzy idea of what these terms mean.

The concepts of yin and yang can be used to describe everything that exists in the universe, including all the parts and functions of the body. Originally, yin referred to the shady side of a hill and yang to the sunny side of the hill. Since sunshine and shade are two, interdependent sides of a single reality, these two aspects of the hill are seen as part of a single whole. Other examples of yin and yang are that night exists only in relation to day and cold exists only in relation to heat. According to Chinese thought, every single thing that exists in the universe has these two aspects, a yin and a yang. Thus everything has a front and a back, a top and a bottom, a left and a right, and a beginning and an end. However, a thing is yin or yang *only in relation to its paired complement*. Nothing is in itself yin or yang.

It is the concepts of yin and yang which make Chinese medicine a holistic medicine. This is because, based on this unitary and complementary vision of reality, no body part or body function is viewed as separate or isolated from the whole person. The table below shows a partial list of yin and yang pairs as they apply to the body.

Yin	Yang
form	function
organs	bowels
blood	qi
inside	outside
front of body	back of body
right side	left side
lower body	upper body
cool, cold	warm, hot
stillness	activity, movement

However, it is important to remember that each item listed is either yin or yang only in relation to its complementary partner. Nothing is absolutely and all by itself either yin or yang. As we can see from the above list, it is possible to describe every aspect of the body in terms of yin and yang.

8

Qi

Qi (pronounced chee) and blood are the two most important complementary pairs of yin and yang within the human body. It is said that, in the world, yin and yang are water and fire, but in the human body, yin and yang are blood and qi. Qi is yang in relation to blood which is yin. Qi is often translated as energy and certainly energy is a manifestation of qi. Chinese language scholars would say, however, that qi is larger than any single type of energy described by modern Western science. Paul Unschuld, perhaps the greatest living Sinologist, translates the word qi as influences. This conveys the sense that qi is what is responsible for change and movement. Thus, within Chinese medicine, qi is that which motivates all movement and transformation or change.

In Chinese medicine, qi is defined as having five specific functions:

1. Defense

It is qi which is responsible for protecting the exterior of the body from invasion by external pathogens. This qi, called defensive qi, flows through the exterior portion of the body.

2. Transformation

Qi transforms substances so that they can be utilized by the body. An example of this function is the transformation of the food we eat into nutrients to nourish the body, thus producing more qi and blood.

3. Warming

Qi, being relatively yang, is inherently warm and one of the main functions of the qi is to warm the entire body, both inside and out. If this warming function of the qi is weak, cold may cause the flow of qi and blood to be congealed similar to cold's effect on water producing ice.

4. Restraint

It is qi which holds all the organs and substances in their proper place. Thus all the organs, blood, and fluids need qi to keep them from falling or leaking out of their specific pathways. If this function of the qi is weak, then problems like uterine prolapse, easy bruising, or urinary incontinence may occur.

5. Transportation

Qi provides the motivating force for all transportation and movement in the body. Every aspect of the body that moves is moved by the qi. Hence the qi moves the blood and body fluids throughout the body. It moves food through the stomach and blood through the vessels.

Blood

In Chinese medicine, blood refers to the red fluid that flows through our vessels the same as in modern Western medicine, but it also has meanings and implications which are different from those in modern Western medicine. Most basically, blood is that substance which nourishes and moistens all the body tissues. Without blood, no body tissue can function properly. In addition, when blood is insufficient or scanty, tissue becomes dry and withers.

Qi and blood are closely interrelated. It is said that, "Qi is the commander of the blood and blood is the mother of qi." This means that it is qi which moves the blood but that it is the blood which provides the nourishment and physical foundation for the creation and existence of the qi.

In Chinese medicine, blood provides the following functions for the body:

1. Nourishment

Blood nourishes the body. Along with qi, the blood goes to every part of the body. When the blood is insufficient, function decreases and tissue atrophies or shrinks.

2. Moistening

Blood moistens the body tissues. This includes the skin, eyes, and ligaments and tendons or what are simply called the sinews in Chinese medicine. Thus blood insufficiency can cause drying out and consequent stiffening of various body tissues throughout the body.

3. Blood provides the material foundation for the spirit or mind.

In Chinese medicine, the mind and body are not two separate things. The spirit is nothing other than a great accumulation of qi. The blood (yin) supplies the material support and nourishment for the spirit (yang) so that it accumulates, becomes bright (i.e., conscious and clever), and stays rooted in the body. If the blood becomes insufficient, the mind can "float," causing problems like insomnia, agitation, and unrest.

Essence

Along with qi and blood, essence is one of the three most important constituents of the body. Essence is the most fundamental, essential material the body utilizes for its growth, maturation, and reproduction. There are two forms of this essence. We inherit essence from our parents and we also produce our own essence from the food we eat, the liquids we drink, and the air we breathe.

The essence which comes from our parents is what determines our basic constitution, strength, and vitality. We each have a finite, limited amount of this inherited essence. It is important to protect and conserve this essence because all bodily functions depend upon it and, when it is gone, we die. Thus the depletion of essence has serious implications for our overall health and well-being. Happily, the essence derived from food and drink helps to bolster and support this inherited essence. Thus, if we eat well and do not consume more qi and blood than we create each day, then when we sleep at night, this surplus qi and more especially blood is transformed into essence.

The Viscera & Bowels

In Chinese medicine, the internal organs (called viscera so as not to become confused with the Western biological entities of the same name) have a wider area of function and influence than in Western medicine. Each viscus has distinct responsibilities for maintaining the physical and psychological health of the individual. When thinking about the internal viscera according to Chinese medicine, it is more accurate to view them as spheres of influence or a network that spreads throughout the body, rather than as a distinct and separate physical organ as described by Western science. This is why the famous German Sinologist, Manfred Porkert, refers to them as orbs rather than as organs. In Chinese medicine, the relationship between the various viscera and other parts of the body is made possible by the channel and network vessel system which we will discuss below.

In Chinese medicine, there are five main viscera which are relatively yin and six main bowels which are relatively yang. The five yin viscera are the heart, lungs, liver, spleen, and kidneys. The six yang bowels are the stomach, small intestine, large intestine, gallbladder, urinary bladder, and a system that Chinese medicine refers to as the triple burner. All the functions of the entire body are subsumed or described under these eleven organs

12

or spheres of influence. Thus Chinese medicine *as a system* does not have a pancreas, a pituitary gland, or the ovaries. Nonetheless, all the functions of these Western organs are described under the Chinese medical system of the five viscera and six bowels.

Within this system, the five viscera are the most important. These are the organs that Chinese medicine says are responsible for the creation and transformation of qi and blood and the storage of essence. For instance, the kidneys are responsible for the excretion of urine but are also responsible for hearing, the strength of the bones, sex, reproduction, maturation and growth, the lower and upper back, and the lower legs in general and the knees in particular.

Visceral Correspondences

Organ	Tissue	Sense	Spirit	Emotion
Kidneys	bones/ head hair	hearing	will	fear
Liver	sinews	sight	ethereal soul	anger
Spleen	flesh	taste	thought	thinking/ worry
Lungs	skin/body hair	smell	corporeal soul	grief/ sadness
Heart	blood vessels	speech	spirit	joy/fright

This points out that the Chinese viscera may have the same name and even some overlapping functions but yet are quite different from the organs of modern Western medicine. Each of the five Chinese medical viscera also has a corresponding tissue, sense, spirit, and emotion related to it. These are outlined in the table above.

In addition, each Chinese medical viscus or bowel possesses both a yin and a yang aspect. The yin aspect of a viscus or bowel refers to its substantial nature or tangible form. Further, an organ's yin is responsible for the nurturing, cooling, and moistening of that viscus or bowel. The yang aspect of the viscus or bowel represents its functional activities or what it does. An organ's yang aspect is also warming. These two aspects, yin and yang, form and function, cooling and heating, when balanced create good health. However, if either yin or yang becomes too strong or too weak, the result will be disease.

The kidneys

In Chinese medicine, the kidneys are considered to be the foundation of our life. Because the developing fetus looks like a large kidney and because the kidneys are the main viscus for the storage of inherited essence, the kidneys are referred to as the prenatal root. Thus keeping the kidney qi strong and kidney yin and yang in relative balance is considered essential to good health and longevity. The basic Chinese medical statements of fact about the kidneys are:

1. The kidneys are considered responsible for human reproduction, development, and maturation.

These are the same functions we used when describing the essence. This is because the essence is stored in the kidneys. Health problems related to reproduction, development, and maturation are considered to be problems of the kidney essence. Excessive sexual activity, drug use, or simple prolonged over-exhaustion can all damage and consume kidney essence. Kidney essence is also consumed by the simple act of aging.

2. The kidneys are the foundation of water metabolism.

The kidneys work in coordination with the lungs and spleen to insure that water is spread properly throughout the body and that

14

excess water is excreted as urination. Therefore, problems such as edema, excessive dryness, or excessive day or nighttime urination can indicate a weakness of kidney function.

3. The kidneys are responsible for hearing since the kidneys open through the portals of the ears.

Therefore, auditory problems such as diminished hearing and ringing in the ears can be due to kidney weakness.

4. The kidneys rule the grasping of qi.

This means that one of the functions of the kidney qi is to pull down or absorb the breath from the lungs and root it in the lower abdomen. Certain types of asthma and chronic cough are the result of a weakness in this kidney function.

5. The kidneys rule the bones and marrow.

This means that problems of the bones, such as osteoporosis, degenerative disc disease, and weak legs and knees, can all reflect a kidney problem.

6. Kidney yin and yang are the foundation for the yin and yang of all the other organs and bowels and body tissues of the entire body.

This is another way of saying that the kidneys are the foundation of our life. If either kidney yin or yang is insufficient, eventually the yin or yang of the other organs will also become insufficient. The clinical implications of this will become more clear when we present low back pain case histories.

7. The kidneys store the will.

If kidney qi is insufficient, this aspect of our human nature can be weakened. Conversely, pushing ourselves to extremes, such as long distance running or cycling, can eventually exhaust our kidneys.

8. Fear is the emotion associated with the kidneys.

This means that fear can manifest when the kidney qi is insufficient. Vice versa, constant or excessive fear can damage the kidneys and make them weak.

9. The low back is the mansion of the kidneys.

This means that, of all the areas of the body, the low back is the most closely related to the health of the kidneys. If the kidneys are weak, then there may be low back pain. It is because of this and the fact that the kidneys are associated with the bones that the kidneys are the first and most important viscus in terms of the health and well-being of the low back according to Chinese medicine.

The liver

In Chinese medicine, the liver is associated with one's emotional state, with digestion, and with menstruation in women. The basic Chinese medical statements of facts concerning the liver include:

1. The liver controls coursing and discharge.

Coursing and discharge refer to the uninhibited spreading of qi to every part of the body. If the liver is not able to maintain the free and smooth flow of qi throughout the body, multiple physical and emotional symptoms can develop. This function of the liver is most easily damaged by emotional causes and, in particular, by anger and frustration. For example, if the liver is stressed due to pent-up anger, the flow of liver qi can become depressed or stagnate.

Liver qi stagnation can cause a wide range of health problems, including PMS, chronic digestive disturbance, depression, and insomnia. Therefore, it is essential to keep our liver qi flowing freely.

2. The liver stores the blood.

This means that the liver regulates the amount of blood in circulation. In particular, when the body is at rest, the blood in the extremities returns to the liver. As an extension of this, it is said in Chinese medicine that the liver is yin in form but yang in function. Thus the liver requires sufficient blood to keep it and its associated tissues moist and supple, cool and relaxed.

3. The liver controls the sinews.

The sinews refer mainly to the tendons and ligaments in the body. Proper function of the tendons and ligaments depends upon the nourishment of liver blood to keep them moist and supple.

4. The liver opens into the portals of the eyes.

The eyes are the specific sense organ corresponding to the liver. Therefore, many eye problems are related to the liver in Chinese medicine.

5. The emotion associated with the liver is anger.

Anger is the emotion that typically arises when the liver is diseased and especially when its qi does not flow freely. Conversely, anger damages the liver. Thus the emotions related to the stagnation of qi in the liver are frustration, anger, and rage.

17

The heart

Although the heart is the emperor of the body-mind according to Chinese medicine, it does not play as large a role in the creation and treatment of disease as one might think. Rather than the emperor initiating the cause of disease, in Chinese medicine, mostly enduring disease eventually affects the heart. Especially in terms of insomnia, disturbances of the heart tend to be secondary rather than primary. By this I mean that first some other viscus or bowel becomes diseased and then the heart feels the negative effect. The basic statements of fact about the heart in Chinese medicine are:

1. The heart governs the blood.

This means that it is the heart qi which "stirs" or moves the blood within its vessels. This is roughly analogous to the heart's pumping the blood in Western medicine. The pulsation of the blood through the arteries due to the contraction of the heart is referred to as the "stirring of the pulse." In fact, the Chinese word for pulse and vessel is the same. So this could also be translated as the "stirring of the vessels."

2. The heart stores the spirit.

The spirit refers to the mind in Chinese medicine. Therefore, this statement underscores that mental function, mental clarity, and mental equilibrium are all associated with the heart. If the heart does not receive enough qi or blood or if the heart is disturbed by something, the spirit may become restless and this may produce symptoms of mental-emotional unrest, heart palpitations, insomnia, profuse dreams, etc.

3. The heart governs the vessels.

This statement is very close to number one above. The vessels refer to the blood vessels and also to the pulse.

4. The heart governs speech.

If heart function becomes abnormal, this may be reflected in various speech problems and especially in raving and delirious speech, muttering to oneself, and speaking incoherently.

5. The heart opens into the portal of the tongue.

Because the heart has a special relationship with the tip of the tongue, heart problems may manifest as sores on the tip of the tongue.

6. Joy is the emotion associated with the heart.

The word joy has been interpreted by both Chinese and Westerners in different ways. On the one hand, joy can mean overexcitation, in which case excessive joy can cause problems with the Chinese medical functions of the heart in terms of governing the blood and storing the spirit. On the other hand, joy may be seen as an antidote to the other six emotions of Chinese medicine. From this point of view, joy causes the flow of qi (and therefore blood) to relax and become more moderate and harmonious. If some other emotion causes the qi to become bound or move chaotically, then joy can make it relax and flow normally and smoothly.

The spleen

The spleen is less important in Western medicine than it is in Chinese medicine. Since at least the Yuan dynasty (1280-1368 CE), the spleen has been one of the two most important viscera of

19

Chinese medicine (the other being the kidneys). In Chinese medicine, the spleen plays a pivotal role in the creation of qi and blood and in the circulation and transformation of body fluids. Therefore, when it comes to the spleen, it is especially important not to think of this Chinese viscus in the same way as the Western spleen. The main statements of fact concerning the spleen in Chinese medicine are:

1. The spleen governs movement and transformation.

This refers to the movement and transformation of foods and liquids through the digestive system. In this case, movement and transformation may be paraphrased as digestion. However, secondarily, movement and transformation also refer to the movement and transformation of body fluids through the body. It is the spleen qi which is largely responsible for controlling liquid metabolism in the body.

2. The spleen restrains the blood.

As mentioned above, one of the five functions of the qi is to restrain the fluids of the body, including the blood, within their proper channels and reservoirs. If the spleen qi is healthy and abundant, then the blood is held within its vessels properly. However, if the spleen qi becomes weak and insufficient, then the blood may flow outside its channels and vessels resulting in various types of pathological bleeding. This includes various types of pathological bleeding associated with the menstrual cycle.

3. The spleen stores the constructive.

The constructive is one of the types of qi in the body. Specifically, it is the qi responsible for nourishing and constructing the body and its tissues. This constructive qi is closely associated with the process of digestion and the creation of qi and blood out of food and liquids. If the spleen fails to store or runs out of constructive qi, then the person becomes hungry on the one hand, and eventually becomes fatigued on the other.

4. The spleen governs the muscles and flesh.

This statement is closely allied to the previous one. It is the constructive qi which constructs or nourishes the muscles and flesh. If there is sufficient spleen qi producing sufficient constructive qi, then the person's body is well fleshed and rounded. In addition, their muscles are normally strong. Conversely, if the spleen becomes weak, this may lead to emaciation and/or lack of strength.

5. The spleen governs the four limbs.

This means that the strength and function of the four limbs is closely associated with the spleen. If the spleen is healthy and strong, then there is sufficient strength in the four limbs and warmth in the four extremities. If the spleen becomes weak and insufficient, then there may be lack of strength in the four limbs, lack of warmth in the extremities, or even tingling and numbness in the extremities.

6. The spleen opens into the portal of the mouth.

Just as the ears are the portals of the kidneys, the eyes are the portal of the liver, and the tongue is the portal of the heart, the mouth is the portal of the spleen. Therefore, spleen disease often manifests as mouth or cankersores or bleeding from the gums.

7. Thought is the emotion associated with the spleen.

In the West, we do not usually think of thought as an emotion per se. Be that as it may, in Chinese medicine it is classified along with anger, joy, fear, grief, and melancholy. In particular, thinking, or perhaps I should say overthinking, causes the spleen qi to bind. This means that the spleen qi does not flow harmoniously and this typically manifests as loss of appetite, abdominal bloating after meals, and indigestion.

8. The spleen is the source of engenderment and transformation.

Engenderment and transformation refer to the creation or production of the qi and blood out of the food and drink we take in each day. If the spleen receives adequate food and drink and then properly transforms that food and drink, it engenders or creates the qi and blood. Although the kidneys and lungs also participate in the creation of the qi, while the kidneys and heart also participate in the creation of the blood, the spleen is the pivotal viscus in both processes, and spleen qi weakness and insufficiency is a leading cause of qi and blood insufficiency and weakness.

The lungs

The lungs are not one of the main Chinese viscera in the cause of insomnia. However, like the heart, the lungs often bear the brunt of disease processes initiated in other viscera and bowels. As in Western medicine, the lungs are often subject to externally invading pathogens resulting in respiratory tract diseases. However, the lungs sphere of influence also includes the skin and fluid metabolism. The main statements of fact regarding the lungs in Chinese medicine are:

1. The lungs govern the qi.

Specifically, the lungs govern the downward spread and circulation of the qi. It is the lung qi which moves all the rest of the qi in the body out to the edges and from the top of the body downward. Thus the lung qi is something like a sprinkler spraying out qi. As an extension of this, this downward qi then makes sure body fluids are moved throughout the body and eventually down to the kidneys and bladder and, eventually, out of the body.

2. The lungs govern the skin and hair.

The skin and body hair correspond with the lungs. If the lungs become diseased, this often manifests as skin problems.

3. The lungs govern the voice.

If there is sufficient lung qi, the voice is strong and clear. If there is insufficient lung qi, then the voice is weak and the person tries not to speak as a way of conserving their energy.

4. The lungs govern the free flow and regulation of the water passageways.

This statement emphasizes the lung qi's role in moving body fluids outward and downward throughout the body, ultimately to arrive at the urinary bladder. If the lung qi fails to maintain the free flow and regulation of the water passageways, then fluids will collect and transform into dampness, thus producing water swelling or edema.

5. The lungs govern the defensive exterior.

We say above that the qi defends the body against invasion by external pathogens. In Chinese medicine, the exterior-most layer of the body is the area where the defensive qi circulates and the place where this defense, therefore, takes place. In particular, it is the lungs which govern this defensive qi. If the lungs function normally and there is sufficient defensive qi, then the body cannot be invaded by external pathogens. If the lungs are weak and the defensive qi is insufficient, then external pathogens may easily invade the exterior of the body, causing complaints such as colds, flus, and allergies.

6. The lungs are the florid canopy.

This means that the lungs are like a tent spreading over the top of all the other viscera and bowels. On the one hand, they are the first viscus to be assaulted by external pathogens invading the body from the top. On the other, any pathogenic qi moving upward in the body eventually may accumulate in and affect the lungs.

7. The lungs are the delicate viscus.

Because the lungs are the most delicate of all the viscera and bowels, they are the most easily invaded by external pathogens. This is the Chinese explanation for the prevalence of colds and flus in comparison to other types of diseases.

8. The lungs form snivel.

This means that snivel or nasal mucus has to do, at least in part, with lung function. If the lungs are functioning correctly, there should not be any runny nose or nasal congestion.

9. The lungs open into the portal of the nose.

This statement is similar to the one above. However, it approaches the issue from a slightly different perspective. The implication of this statement is that diseases having to do with the nose and its function are often associated with the Chinese medical idea of the lungs.

Each yin viscus is paired with a yang bowel in a yin-yang or exterior-interior relationship. The kidneys are paired with the urinary bladder, the liver is paired with the gallbladder, the heart is paired with the small intestine, the spleen is paired with the stomach, and the lungs are paired with the large intestine. The yin viscus is relatively more interior and the yang bowel is relatively more exterior. In the case of the urinary bladder, gallbladder, and stomach, these bowels receive their qi from their paired viscus and function very much as an extension of that viscus. The relationship between the other two viscera and bowels is not as close.

In terms of insomnia, Chinese medical theory only concerns itself with two of the six bowels. These are the gallbladder and the stomach.

The gallbladder

The main statements of fact concerning the gallbladder in terms of insomnia in Chinese medicine are:

1. The gallbladder governs decision.

In Chinese medicine, the liver is likened to a general who plans strategy for the body, while the gallbladder is likened to a judge. According to this point of view, if a person lacks gallbladder qi, they will have trouble making decisions. In addition, they will be timid. While courage in the West is associated with the heart (*coeur* = courage), bravery in the East is associated with the gallbladder. Actually, this is also an old Western idea as well. When someone is very forward and brazen, we say that "They have gall." Conversely, if someone is excessively timid, this may be due to gallbladder qi vacuity or insufficiency. In Chinese medicine, this is called "gallbladder timidity."

2. The liver and gallbladder have the same palace.

This statement underscores the particularly close relationship between the liver and gallbladder.

3. If there is qi because of a robust gallbladder, evils are not able to enter.

These two statements are very close to statements in Chinese medicine about the heart saying that the heart is the sovereign of the body and that if spirit abides (in the heart), then evils cannot enter. Both these statements elevate the gallbladder to a place of importance in the body it does not hold in Western medicine and link the gallbladder in a way to the heart and its spirit.

The stomach

There are a number of important statements of fact concerning the stomach in Chinese medicine due to the stomach's pivotal role in digestion and, therefore, in the creation of qi and blood. Below we will only discuss those statements which we will use later in our discussion of the disease causes and disease mechanisms of insomnia in Chinese medicine.

1. The stomach governs intake.

This means that the stomach is the first to receive foods and drinks ingested into the body.

2. The stomach governs downbearing of the turbid.

The process of digestion in Chinese medicine is likened to the process of fermentation and then distillation. The stomach is the fermentation tun wherein foods and liquids are "rottened and ripened." This rottening and ripening allows for the separation of clear and turbid parts of the digestate. The spleen sends the clear parts upward to the lungs and heart to become the qi and blood respectively. The stomach's job is to send the turbid part down to be excreted as waste from the large intestine and bladder.

3. Stomach heat may exploit the heart.

If, for any reason, abnormal or pathological heat collects in the stomach, because heat is yang and has an innate tendency to move upward and outward, and because the heart is located above the stomach in Chinese medicine, heat in the stomach may exploit or harass the heart above.

4. The stomach is the origin of the defensive qi.

We have seen above that the defensive qi is the qi which defends the exterior of the body from invasion by external pathogens. This defensive qi's other job is to warm the internal organs. According to some points of view, the stomach is the origin of the defensive qi. This is because it is in the stomach that the clear and turbid parts of the digestate are separated, and the defensive qi is made out of a further refinement of the turbid part of this digestate. Therefore, the stomach has a definite relationship with the defensive qi, and, as we will see below, this relationship can help explain at least one type of insomnia.

Above I mentioned that there are five viscera and six bowels. The sixth bowel is called the triple burner. It is said in Chinese that, "The triple burner has a function but no form." The name triple burner refers to the three main areas of the torso. The upper burner is the chest. The middle burner is the space from the bottom of the ribcage to the level of the navel. The lower burner is the lower abdomen below the navel. These three spaces are called burners because all of the functions and transformations of the viscera and bowels which they contain as "warm" trans-formations similar to food cooking in a pot on a stove or similar to an alchemical transformation in a furnace. In fact, the triple burner is nothing other than a generalized concept of how the other viscera and bowels function together as an organic unit in terms of the digestion of foods and liquids and the circulation and transformation of body fluids.

The Channels & Network Vessels

Each viscus and bowel has a corresponding channel with which it is connected. In Chinese medicine, the inside of the body is made up of the viscera and bowels. The outside of the body is composed of the sinews and bones, muscles and flesh, and skin and hair. It is the channels and network vessels (*i.e.*, smaller connecting vessels) which connect the inside and the outside of the body. It is through these channels and network vessels that the viscera and bowels connect with their corresponding body tissues.

The channels and network vessel system is a unique feature of traditional Chinese medicine. These channels and vessels are different from the circulatory, nervous, or lymphatic systems. The earliest reference to these channels and vessels is in *Nei Jing (Inner Classic)*, a text written around the 2nd or 3rd century BCE.

The channels and vessels perform two basic functions. They are the pathways by which the qi and blood circulate through the body and between the organs and tissues. Additionally, as mentioned above, the channels connect the viscera and bowels internally with the exterior part of the body. This channel and vessel system functions in the body much like the world information communication network. The channels allow the various parts of our body to cooperate and interact to maintain our lives.

This channel and network vessel system is complex. There are 12 primary channels, 6 yin and 6 yang, each with a specific pathway through the external body and connected with an internal organ (see diagrams below). There are also extraordinary vessels, sinew channels, channel divergences, main network vessels, and ultimately countless finer and finer network vessels permeating the entire body. All of these form a closed loop or circuit similar to but distinct from the Western circulatory system.

28

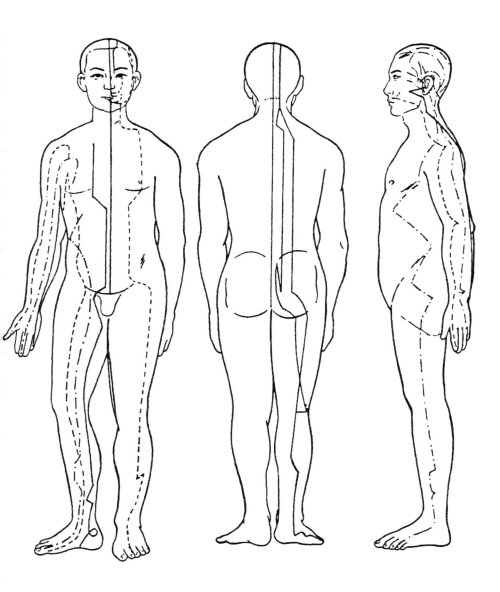

Acupuncture points are places located on the major channels where there is a special concentration of qi and blood. Because of the relatively more qi and blood accumulated at these places, the sites act as switches which can potentially control the flow of qi and blood in the channel on which the point is located. By stimulating these points in any of a number of different ways, one can speed up or slow down, make more or reduce, warm or cool down the qi and blood flowing in the channels and vessels. The main ways of stimulating these points and thus adjusting the flow of qi and blood in the channels and vessels is to needle them and to heat them by moxibustion.[2] Other commonly used ways of stimulating these points and thus adjusting the qi and blood flowing through the channels and vessels are massage, cupping, the application of magnets, and the application of various herbal medicinals. If the channels and vessels are the pathways over which the qi and blood flow, then the acupuncture points are the places where this flow can be adjusted.

---

[2] Moxibustion refers to adding heat to an acupuncture point or area of the body by burning a dried herb, Folium Artemisae Argyii (*Ai Ye*), Oriental Mugwort, on, over, or near the area to be warmed.

Sleep & Wakefulness in Chinese Medicine

Sleep and wakefulness are a yin-yang pair in Chinese medicine. Consciousness is called *shen ming* in Chinese medicine. *Shen* means the spirit, while *ming* means brightness or brilliance. In addition, the spirit is nothing other than an accumulation of yang qi in the heart. In the closing to his monumental *Pi Wei Lun (Treatise on the Spleen & Stomach)*, Li Dong-yuan, one of the four great masters of medicine of the Jin-Yuan dynasties (1280-1368 CE), explained the relationship between the spirit, qi, and essence thus:

> Qi is the forefather of spirit and essence is the child of qi. (Therefore,) qi is the root of essence and spirit. Great is qi!

When yang qi ascends to the upper body to accumulate in the heart as spirit and to the sensory orifices of the head as clear yang qi, the mind is awake and the senses are conscious. The eyes and ears are open and functioning and the person is "conscious of human affairs."

Clear yang qi is produced out of the food and drink we take in each day as well as the air we breathe. It is the clear part of food and drink sent up to the lungs by the spleen which combines with the heavenly or great qi breathed in by the lungs which becomes the constructive qi which empowers, nourishes, and constructs the body.

Sleep, on the other hand, is the sinking of this clear yang qi back downward and into the core of the body to be "enfolded" and

31

nurtured by yin. The yang qi sinks back downward and into the core of the body because it has been consumed by the day's activities. In other words, the processes of seeing, hearing, smelling, tasting, thinking, moving, emoting, and all other life processes use up yang qi in the course of their activity. When we have used up a certain sufficiency of yang qi, we no longer have enough to keep our spirit bright and in contact with the outer world. During sleep, yin blood nourishes and transforms into yang qi. Thus when our yang qi has recuperated after a number of hours of sleep, we wake back up again, ready to face the challenges and activities of a new day.

The fact our body's yang qi comes upward and outward around daybreak and retreats back downward and inward after the sun goes down is due to our body's qi being influenced by the larger qi of the external universe. The sun is called *tai yang* or supreme yang in Chinese. Its rising each morning is seen as a growth of yang qi in the world at large. At noon, this yang qi reaches its extreme and begins to descend and retreat again. Therefore, the ruling qi of day is yang which grows from sunup to noon and declines from noon to sundown, while the ruling qi of night is yin which grows from sundown to midnight and declines from midnight to sunup. Thus the body's yin and yang also follows suit. It is said in Chinese medicine, "Humans exist within heaven and earth and, therefore, correspond (*i.e.*, co-respond or resonate) with the sun and moon."

The rate of consumption each day of our yang qi and the blood and yin which support and nourish it is dependent upon and proportional to each day's activities. When we are more active, we consume more yang qi. When we are less active, we consume less yang qi. Therefore, on days when we work harder, we may feel more tired more quickly than on other days. Hence, we may want to go to sleep earlier and/or sleep longer. If, for some reason, we cannot go to sleep when we want to, we begin to consume even more qi (and blood) than usual. If we consume all the qi and blood which we manufactured that day, then we start dipping into our reserves. These reserves are the essence that is stored in each of the five viscera but whose major portion is stored in the kidneys. When push comes to shove or when the going gets tough and the tough get going, stored essence is tranformed into qi. From this point of view, essence is yin to qi's yang and yin essence may be transformed into yang qi.

If one has plenty of stored essence, then this is no big deal. The next day, if one eats and drinks right and one's lungs are functioning correctly, and if one's activities do not use up all the qi and blood manufactured that day, then the surplus that is left over when we go to sleep the next night is converted back into stored essence.

Age & sleep

When we are babies, it is axiomatic in Chinese medicine that our viscera and bowels are immature and that our qi and blood are not plentiful and robust. Therefore, newborns mostly sleep all day and wake only for short periods to eat. Their immature viscera and bowels simply do not produce enough qi and blood to keep the newborn's yang qi in the upper and outer part of his or her body for any length of time. As the child grows, their viscera and bowels mature. This means that they become more and more efficient in transforming qi and blood out of the food they eat and the air they breathe.

When we are a young adult, if A) we have a normal constitution, B) we are eating a relatively healthy diet, and C) we are not grossly overtaxing ourselves each day, we each make plenty more qi and blood each day than we consume. Therefore, we make plenty of new essence to be stored in the five viscera and especially the kidneys. As, when we are young, we may overwork one day, but the next be bright-eyed and bushy-tailed again. Or

33

we may "pull an all-nighter" in college and the next day be none the worse for wear.

Mostly, this superabundance of qi and blood and, therefore, of acquired essence is due to the spleen's maturation at around six years of age. It is said that the spleen is the postnatal root of qi and blood engenderment and transformation. This is because it is the spleen which is in charge of transforming or refining the pure or clear part of the digestate to become the qi and blood. Hence, the sufficiency of qi and blood and, consequently, acquired essence is primarily dependent upon a healthy spleen processing sufficient nutrition. If either the spleen is not given the raw materials to transform or if the spleen qi is not capable of doing its duty, qi and blood production will not be up to par.

It is said in the *Nei Jing (The Inner Classic)*, the so-called Bible of Chinese medicine written some 2200 years ago, that the digestion begins to decline at around 35 years of age. Because of this, the spleen does not make as much blood, and because there is not as much blood to nourish and moisten the skin, one begins to get wrinkles on their face. This clearly underscores that the aging process begins with the decline of the process of digestion and the manufacture of qi and blood, and this process of digestion is governed and primarily based on the Chinese medical concept of the spleen.

This is also the explanation why we typically need more sleep and tire more easily after 35 years of age. We may look at our younger sisters and brothers in the full bloom of their 20s, carousing all night and getting up for work the next morning, and wonder how they do it. They do it because their spleen's are still manufacturing so much qi and blood every day. However, past 35, we no longer make the same superabundance of qi and blood and start drawing down on the yin essence stored in our kidneys.

This then further means that the aging process in humans has to do with the consumption of yin by yang. Yang is active and consumes yin, but, after a certain age, we no longer replace and replenish the yin we are using up. Therefore, the aging process is, at least in part, a process of drying up (since yin is cool and moist). Wrinkles, greying of the hair, falling teeth, falling hair, and osteoporsis are all manifestations of the consumption and non-replacement of yin substance by yang function.

At first, decrease in qi and blood due to aging may make us more easily fatigued and prompt us to go to bed earlier and sleep longer. However, it is a basic tenet of yin-yang theory that yin checks or controls yang. If yin becomes so vacuous and weak that it cannot control yang, then yang may counterflow upward and outward. This upward and outward flow of yang is not a healthy movement. Yang is not rising upward because there is a true superabundance of clear yang qi. Rather, it is rising up when it shouldn't because there is insufficient yin to hold it down. This explains why so many people develop matitudinal insomnia as they age. Yang qi runs out of steam at the end of the day and initially they go to sleep. But there is insufficient yin to enfold and hold yang down for long. Yang is relatively out of balance from yin, and so, as soon as the sun, *tai yang* begins to move upward in the world outside, our own yang, also pops back up out of control too early in the AM.

Therefore, anything which stirs yang qi to move upward and outward may cause or aggravate insomnia, and we will look at some of the specific causes of this below. Some readers may, at this point, be thinking that, since consumption of yin is an inevitable part of aging, that, past a certain age, there is nothing that can be done about insomnia. However, as we see below, Chinese medicine has simple, safe, and effective ways of stimulating the body to produce more blood and yin, *thus actually slowing down the aging process.*

The uterus & sleep

To the uninitiated, the above header must seem very strange. What does the uterus have to do with sleep? In Chinese medicine, it is said that men and women are essentially the same *except that women have a uterus*. Because they have a uterus, they menstruate, can have babies, and lactate. According to Chinese medicine, this makes women more prone to insomnia, at least at certain times, than men are.

Menstruation is a discharge or loss of blood each month, and blood is part of yin. In fact, the famous Qing dynasty (1644-1911 CE) Chinese gynecologist, Fu Qing-zhu, said that the menstrual blood in women should not just be seen as blood but as the physical expression of their yin essence. When a woman is young and in good health, she makes a superabundance of blood each month and this superabundance is discharged as the menses. Because she is making so much qi and blood in turn due to her strong, healthy spleen, this blood loss causes no problem. However, in women with weak spleens or in many women as they age, they may experience insomnia each month either before, during, or right after their menstruation. If a woman's blood is scanty, when that blood is sent down by the heart to accumulate in the uterus in the premenstruum, she may not have enough yin blood left over to control yang qi. This yang qi counterflows upward and outward, manifesting as insomnia or wakefulness. Or perhaps, she has enough blood so that yin controls yang during the premenstruum but not enough blood to control yang once she starts to actually lose blood with the menstrual flow. In this case, the woman may develop insomnia during or after her menses when it is said her blood is relatively empty.

Likewise, some women develop insomnia either during pregnancy or after delivery. In Chinese medicine, the baby's body is made out of the mother's essence and blood. Towards the end of the pregnancy when the baby has grown so big, some women will have used up so much blood and essence that their yin can no longer control their yang. In other cases, some women will lose so much blood and sweat during labor or with their postpartum lochia or vaginal discharge that now their yin is insufficient to control yang. And because breast milk is made out of the mother's blood according to Chinese medicine, women whose blood and yin are scanty to begin with often experience worsening of this yin vacuity during breast-feeding. This is why some women may develop insomnia associated with breast-feeding.

And finally, women in particular are prone to insomnia around the time of menopause. The pause in menstruation occurs because the body in its wisdom recognizes that it can no longer support in a healthy manner either a monthly loss of blood during menstruation nor another pregnancy. From the mid-30s onward, most women will notice their menses become progressively less voluminous. This goes along with a decrease in blood production in turn due to a decrease in spleen function associated with aging. As the woman gets into her 40s, she is not making sufficient blood to afford a monthly menstruation. This monthly loss of blood in many women actually causes a yin insufficiency and a relative yang excess or repletion. This is why many women develop insomnia around the time of menopause. It is due to the relationship of blood and essence and essence and yin. Hence, in Chinese medicine, we recognize that women, due to "having a uterus," are at special risk for suffering from insomnia, either at certain times of the month or at certain times of their lives.

The Chinese Mechanisms of Insomnia

Now that we've gone over basic Chinese medical theory and discussed sleep and wakefulness from the Chinese point of view, we can look at the specific causes and mechanisms of insomnia identified in Chinese medicine.

Disease causes & disease mechanisms

There are eight basic causes and mechanisms of insomnia in Chinese medicine. Each of these causes leads to an imbalance of yin and yang in the body. Yin fails to control yang, and, therefore, yang counterflows upward and outward.

1. Heart-spleen dual vacuity

Heart-spleen dual vacuity may also be called heart blood-spleen qi vacuity. If thinking, worry, overtaxation, or fatigue are excessive, any of these may damage the spleen. Because the spleen is the root of qi and blood engenderment and trans-formation, spleen qi which is vacuous and weak will fail to manufacture and send up enough blood to the heart spirit. Spirit is nothing other than an accumulation of yang qi. If the heart does not receive sufficient blood to nourish and control this spirit, the heart spirit will grow restless and lose its tranquility. Hence it cannot subside and be enfolded by and in yin at night. In Chinese medicine, the day is yang compared to the night being yin. Therefore, during the day, yang qi is preeminent in the body, while at night, yin blood is preeminent within the human organism. Because the role of the blood is preeminent at night, if yin blood is scanty and insufficient, it tends to manifest this all the more strongly at night. As one ancient Chinese medical text puts, it: "If thinking and worry damage the spleen and spleen blood becomes debilitated and suffers detriment, insomnia may continue for years."

It is interesting to note that thinking here simply means the process of thinking itself. It's ill effect does not depend on whether one's thoughts are good or bad. Thinking is a yang activity of the spirit which consumes yin blood. If thinking is excessive, then there will be excessive consumption of yin blood.

Although Chinese medical texts tend to emphasize the negative role of overthinking and too much work, too little exercise and faulty diet may also contribute to a heart-spleen vacuity. While too much work or exercise overly consumes the qi and blood manufactured by the spleen, too little exercise causes the qi mechanism to become stagnant. The qi mechanism is the mechanism of upbearing the pure or clear part of the digestate and downbearing the turbid part. This upbearing and downbearing is dependent on the free and active flow of qi. When one fails to get sufficient exercise, the qi does not flow smoothly and freely, and so upbearing and downbearing and the consequent engenderment and transformation of qi and blood is also sluggish and insufficient.

In addition, eating the wrong foods may also damage the spleen, thus resulting in a heart blood vacuity. As we will see below, the process of digestion is a warm transformation of yang qi working on and refining yin substance. Therefore, eating too many chilled and uncooked foods and drinking iced liquids can douse the digestive fire of the spleen. Likewise, eating too many sugars and sweets may also damage the spleen. This includes too many sweet and juicy fruits and fruit juices, like oranges and peaches. And finally, eating too many dairy products and fatty foods may damage the spleen, leading to spleen vacuity and consequent qi and blood vacuity.

2. Liver depression qi stagnation

As we have seen above, the liver's main job is to govern the coursing and discharge of all the qi in the body. This means that it is the liver's job to ensure that the flow of qi is smooth and freely flowing. If a person's desires are thwarted, this is equivalent to a thwarting of their flow of qi which cannot "spread freely." This frustration in turn affects the liver's coursing and discharging of the qi. Proportional to the frustration, the liver's coursing and discharging of the qi will become depressed and the qi flow stagnant. This is called liver depression qi stagnation. It is mostly due to stress and frustration or a thwarting of one's desires. Because no adult can fulfill all one's desires at the very moment we desire them, most adults suffer from some element of liver depression qi stagnation—the more stress and frustration, the more liver depression and qi stagnation.

In actual fact, liver depression qi stagnation due to emotional stress and frustration does not cause insomnia all by itself. However, if the liver becomes depressed, this typically leads to the spleen becoming vacuous and weak. This is because the liver "controls" the spleen according to an ancient Chinese theory called five phase theory. Based on this theory, the spleen is usually the first viscus to subsequently become diseased after the liver becomes depressed. If the spleen becomes vacuous and weak, it will not engender and transform the qi and blood properly, and this then may lead to a heart blood and spleen qi dual vacuity. In that case, heart blood is too vacuous to nourish and quiet the spirit. The spirit, which is nothing other than an accumulation of yang qi, becomes hyperactive or restless, and this restlessness manifests as wakefulness.

41

It's is also possible for liver depression qi stagnation to lead to yin vacuity. The qi is what moves yin blood to nourish all the viscera and bowels of the body. As it is said in Chinese medicine:

If the qi moves, the blood moves. If the qi stops, the blood stops.

If the qi does not flow freely, the blood and yin cannot flow freely to nourish the viscera and bowels. Hence, long-term or enduring liver depression qi stagnation eventually wind up causing concomitant yin vacuity. In that case, yin fails to control yang which flushes upward and outward causing wakefulness. Since yin tends to become vacuous after the age of 35 or 40 in any case, the negative effects of liver depression depriving the viscera of sufficient nourishment by the blood and yin tend to become more apparent after this age. In Chinese medicine it is said, "Yin is half consumed by 40 years of age."

3. Liver depression transforming heat

There is a theory in Chinese medicine called the theory of similar transformation. Because the body's living qi is yang, and therefore warm in nature, if anything causes this qi to back up and accumulate, it may cause such depressed and stagnant yang qi to transform into or manifest as pathological heat. Therefore, it is said in Chinese medicine that enduring liver depression due to emotional stress and frustration may transform into heat or fire. This is called transformative or depressive heat. This transformation may also take place in a shorter period of time if frustration and stress give way to outright anger and emotional upsetment. It is said in Chinese medicine that, "Any of the seven emotions may transform into fire if extreme."

Fire is by nature yang and, therefore, tends to move upward and outward in the body, drafting along with it the body's host yang qi. In addition, this fire tends to collect in the upper part of the body and the heart. Due to this pathological heat accumulating in

42

the heart, it causes the spirit to flit around restlessly. Could you fall asleep if your house were on fire?

This tendency of depressive heat due to stress and frustration or anger and emotional upsetment to rise up and accumulate in the heart can be aggravated by eating hot, acrid, peppery foods. This includes chilies and peppers, but also greasy, fried, fatty foods, and alcohol. Overeating any of these can give rise to stomach heat which flares upward to accumulate in the heart.

Because heat or fire is yang, it not only moves upward and outward in the body but also evaporates and consumes blood and yin. As we age, because yin is already being consumed, there is, therefore, a tendency for depression to transform into heat even more easily.

4. Yin vacuity, fire effulgence

If, for any reason, yin becomes truly vacuous and insufficient, yang may become hyperactive. If yang becomes very hyperactive, it is called internal fire. Since yin is primarily associated with the kidneys and hyperactive yang is primarily associated with the liver, this is also referred to as kidney yin vacuity with ascendant hyperactivity of liver yang or liver yang harassing and stirring above. Such a kidney yin vacuity may be due to constitutional insufficiency, meaning that the person was simply not born with much yin to begin with. People with very thin bodies tend to suffer from constitutional yin vacuity. Such yin vacuity can be due to aging as we have already seen. Such yin vacuity may also be due to long-term or severe disease and especially a febrile or feverish disease. In that case, the pathological heat associated with the disease consumes and wastes the body's yin blood. Tuberculosis, or what is still called vacuity consumption in Chinese medicine, is a good example of this mechanism.

It is also possible for yin vacuity to be due to simply too much stirring or activity. In Chinese, the word *dong* means to stir. In the Jin-Yuan dynasties, Zhu Dan-xi, the last of the four great doctors of that era, said that, in human beings in general, "Yang tends to be superabundant, while yin is typically insufficient" and that any activity may cause stirring of yang and further consumption of yin. By activity, Zhu meant any physical, mental, or emotional activity. Zhu saw all these activities as manifestations of stirring yang which consumes yin and leads to only more stirring of yang.

In particular, Zhu singled out what, in Chinese, is referred to as "bedroom taxation." Simply put, this means too much sex, and both men and women can suffer from it. Sexual desire in Chinese medicine is a preeminent manifestation of stirring yang. When we are filled with sexual desire, we say we are "hot" with desire. We are all "stirred up." We are "hot and bothered." And we need to take a cold shower to douse "the flames of our desire." All these colloquialisms point to the same truth that the Chinese have known for centuries. In Chinese medicine, sexual desire and sexual activity are both a function of kidney fire or kidney yang. If sexual desire is not fulfilled, then this fire is stirred up and then depressed. This leads to liver depression transforming heat. If the desire is fulfilled, this leads to consumption and loss of yin. In either case, too much desire or too much sex can lead to or worsen yin vacuity with its attendant loss of control over yang.

Likewise, anything which speeds up the body or pushes the body to prolonged excessive activity may lead to yin vacuity and yang hyperactivity. Things which speed up the body are caffeinated drinks, such as coffee, and recreational drugs, such as cocaine and amphetamines (or speed). Prolonged, excessive stirring refers to prolonged, excessive emotions or prolonged excessive activity, such as too much exercise. Any of these can waste yin and stir yang hyperactively. In our modern context, this includes "sex, drugs, and rock n' roll."

If yin becomes extremely vacuous and yang fire becomes extremely hyperactive, yin and yang may come apart and fail to interact in a harmonious and healthy way. Since water is yin and the kidneys are the water viscus according to five phase theory, an ancient system of reciprocal correspondence in Chinese medicine, while fire is yang and the heart is the fire viscus, such an extreme coming apart of yin and yang is sometimes referred to as heart and kidneys not interacting.

5. Heart vacuity & gallbladder timidity[3]

This mechanism of insomnia is often seen in women who are somewhat overweight. Fat or adipose tissue is seen as abnormally accumulated phlegm, dampness, and turbidity in Chinese medicine. Mostly, this is due to a spleen which is too weak to transform the digestate properly. The clear and turbid are not separated completely and turbid dampness lingers, accumulates, and congeals into phlegm. Because the spleen qi is weak, the blood is not produced sufficiently to nourish the heart spirit which becomes restless. Also because the spleen qi is weak and insufficient, heart and lung qi are vacuous and weak. At the same time, due to emotional stress (and in Western culture, being overweight is itself a cause of stress and frustration), there is liver depression qi stagnation. When depressed qi accumulates, because it is yang, it tends to counterflow upward. When it counterflows upward, it may draft phlegm along with it and this phlegm may confound or obstruct the orifices or portals of the heart. When such phlegm causes blockage of the flow of qi and blood to the heart, the spirit becomes even more upset and tends to stir frenetically like a drowning man gasping for air.

---

[3] In China, bravery is associated with the gallbladder. Because timidity and frightfulness are main symptoms of this pattern, it is called gallbladder timidity. However, it is the heart qi which is vacuous and weak and the liver qi which is depressed.

45

Thus this type of insomnia is due to a combination of weak spleen function resulting in heart vacuity on the one hand and phlegm accumulation on the other plus emotional stress resulting in liver depression qi stagnation. While this type of insomnia is mostly seen in women with a tendency to obesity, it is definitely aggravated by faulty diet and by additional stress. Any food or drink which either damages the spleen or gives rise to even more phlegm and dampness will make this disease mechanism worse, as will any emotional stress or frustration making the person's liver more depressed and qi more stagnant.

6. Phlegm fire harassing the heart

This mechanism is essentially the same as the one above. However, in this case, depression has endured long enough or is severe enough for liver depression to turn into depressive heat or fire. Thus there is phlegm blocking the orifices of the heart at the same time as there is fire disturbing the heart spirit. Since the heart spirit is restless, yang qi cannot stop stirring and sinks downward and into the enfolding womb of dark yin. Such depressive heat and phlegm are both aggravated by greasy, fatty fried foods, hot, acrid, peppery foods, and alcohol. This is in addition to the emotional upset which causes liver depression and the faulty diet which damages the spleen and promotes the engenderment of phlegm and dampness.

7. Stomach disharmony

It is also possible for simple overeating to cause insomnia. Typically, this type of insomnia is episodic and secondary to a particular meal which was too large and too late in the day. Food is yin and yin substance can hinder or block the free flow of yang. We have seen above that yang qi follows a daily diurnal cycle of moving upward and outward with the sun in the AM and downward and inward with the sun in the PM. The defensive qi is part of the yang qi in the body and it is this yang qi which is

46

responsible for wakefulness. For sleep to come, the yang qi of the body, including the defensive qi, must travel to the deep interior of the body, away from the surface. If the stomach is full of solid, yin food, the diurnal retreat of defensive yang away from the surface and upper parts of the body is blocked. In this case, the food in the stomach may literally block the yang qi from entering the interior of the body. Remember that the stomach which is a bowel is more "exterior" than the viscera which are yin. If the yang qi gets hung up in the stomach, it is still in a relatively yang part of the body and so there is still consciousness. There is also probably a stomachache! Or at least abdominal fullness.

8. Blood stasis

The Chinese word for stasis is derived from the Chinese word for silt. Therefore, static blood is seen as a kind of dry, dead, or wrecked blood which silts up and, hence, obstructs the channels and vessels. Such blood stasis may be due to traumatic injury, long-standing liver depression qi stagnation failing to move the blood, qi vacuity failing to push the blood, cold congealing the blood, or insufficient blood to nourish the vessels and keep them open and functioning correctly. In Chinese medicine, it is a given that static blood hinders the creation of new or fresh blood. This means that blood stasis may give rise to blood vacuity and blood vacuity may give rise to blood stasis. Although no Chinese texts on insomnia list blood stasis as one of the mechanisms of insomnia, since blood vacuity may fail to nourish the heart spirit and since blood vacuity may lead to yin vacuity with attendant ascendant hyperactivity of yang and heat or fire, blood stasis may complicate many cases of insomnia, especially in women who often have blood stasis in their uterus. Such female blood stasis in the uterus is usually due to enduring liver depression qi stagnation not moving the blood in turn due to emotional stress and frustration or to the after-effects of certain medications and procedures, such as oral birth control pills, abortions, tubal ligations, and pelvic inflammatory disease treated by antibiotics alone.

As the reader can see, in Chinese medicine, there are different causes and mechanisms for insomnia in different people. Some of the causes are age and body type related. Some have to do with mental-emotional causes and reactions. Some have to do with either too much or too little exercise and activity. Some may be due to other diseases in the body. Yet others may be due to faulty diet. Since not all people's insomnia is the same, no one treatment will be effective for everyone. More importantly, if one can identify their pattern of insomnia, one can immediately know what they as individuals should and should not do, eat or not eat. Further, because just the right treatment is given to the right individual, there is healing without side effects or doctor-caused complications.

The Chinese Medical Treatment of Insomnia

The hallmark of professional Chinese medicine is what is known as "treatment based on pattern discrimination." Modern Western medicine bases its treatment on a disease diagnosis. This means that two patients diagnosed as suffering from the same disease will get the same treatment. Traditional Chinese medicine also takes the patient's disease diagnosis into account. However, the choice of treatment is not based on the disease so much as it is on what is called the patient's pattern, and it is treatment based on pattern discrimination which is what makes Chinese medicine the holistic, safe, and effective medicine it is.

In order to explain the difference between a disease and a pattern, let us take headache for example. Everyone who is diagnosed as suffering from a headache has to, by definition, have some pain in their head. In modern Western medicine and other medical systems which primarily prescribe on the basis of a disease diagnosis, one can talk about "headache medicines." However, amongst headache sufferers, one may be a man and the other a woman. One may be old and the other young. One may be fat and the other skinny. One may have pain on the right side of her head and the other may have pain on the left. In one case, the pain may be throbbing and continuous, while the other person's pain may be very sharp but intermittent. In one case, they may also have indigestion, a tendency to loose stools, lack of warmth in their feet, red eyes, a dry mouth and desire for cold drinks, while the other person has a wet, weeping, crusty skin rash with red borders, a tendency to hay fever, ringing in their ears, and dizziness when they stand up. In Chinese medicine just as in modern Western medicine, both these patients suffer from headache. That is their disease diagnosis. However, they also suffer from a whole host of other complaints, have very different types of headaches, and very different constitutions, ages, and sex. In Chinese medicine, the patient's pattern is made up from all these other signs and symptoms and other information. Thus, in Chinese medicine, the pattern describes *the totality of the person as a unique individual*. And in Chinese medicine, treatment is designed to rebalance that entire pattern of imbalance as well as address the major complaint or disease. Thus, there is a saying in Chinese medicine:

One disease, different treatments
Different diseases, same treatment

This means that, in Chinese medicine, two patients with the same named disease diagnosis may receive different treatments *if their Chinese medical patterns are different*, while two patients diagnosed with different named diseases may receive the same treatment *if their Chinese medical pattern is the same*. In other words, in Chinese medicine, treatment is predicated primarily on one's pattern discrimination, not on one's named disease diagnosis. Therefore, each person is treated individually.

Since every patient gets just the treatment which is right to restore balance to their particular body, there are also no unwanted side effects. Side effects come from forcing one part of the body to behave while causing an imbalance in some other part. The medicine may have fit part of the problem but not the entirety of the patient as an individual. This is like robbing Peter to pay Paul. Since Chinese medicine sees the entire body (and mind!) as a single, unified whole, curing imbalance in one area of the body while causing it in another is unacceptable.

Below is a description of the major Chinese medical patterns at work in insomnia.

Treatment based on pattern discrimination

Liver depression qi stagnation

Main symptoms: Irritability, premenstrual breast distention and pain, chest and side of the rib pain, lower abdominal distention and pain, discomfort in the stomach and epigastrium, diminished appetite, possible delayed menstruation whose amount is either scanty or profuse, darkish, stagnant menstrual blood, the menses unable to come easily, a normal or slightly dark tongue with thin, white fur, and a bowstring,[4] fine pulse

Treatment principles: Course the liver and rectify the qi

In actual fact, this pattern by itself does not cause insomnia and it also rarely occurs in the simple, textbook way presented above. However, it is rare to find a patient with insomnia who does not have at least an element of liver depression, and, in such cases, it is important to remedy this condition. Because of a reciprocal relationship between the liver and spleen, when the liver gets depressed, the spleen tends to become vacuous and damp at the same time as the stomach tends to become hot and dry. Because the spleen engenders and transforms the blood, liver depression with spleen vacuity often gives rise to blood vacuity as well. If this pattern endures or due to aggravating circumstances, such as

---

[4] There are 28 main pulse types in Chinese medicine, the bowstring pulse being one of these. It feels like its name implies—like a taut violin or bowstring.

aging, menstruation, or lactation, it may also evolve into liver depression with yin vacuity failing to nourish the viscera, meaning primarily failing to nourish the heart viscus and the spirit the heart houses within it.

Liver depression transforms heat

Main symptoms: All the above signs and symptoms plus the following differences. First, the patient is not just irritable, they are downright angry. Secondly, there is a bitter taste in their mouth in the mornings when they wake. And third, there is yellow tongue fur and a bowstring, *rapid* pulse.

Treatment principles: Course the liver and rectify the qi, clear heat and resolve depression

As we have seen above, this pattern may on its own cause insomnia.

Heart-spleen dual vacuity

Main symptoms: Heart palpitations either before or after the menses or prompted or worsened by exercise and fatigue, loss of sleep, lassitude of the spirit, lack of strength, a slightly puffy face, the amount of the menses either profuse or scanty but pale in color, a pale tongue with thin, white fur, and a soggy, small or fine, weak pulse

Treatment principles: Supplement and nourish heart and spleen qi and blood

Heart-spleen dual vacuity means heart blood vacuity and spleen qi vacuity. If heart blood is more vacuous, the amount of the menstruate is scanty. If spleen qi vacuity is more prominent, the amount of discharge is profuse. However, in both cases, the color of the menstruate tends to be pale. Likewise, if the spleen is vacuous and, therefore, also damp, the pulse will be soggy.[5] But if blood is vacuous, the pulse will be fine. As with the above pattern, this one also is rarely if ever seen in its simple, discrete form in clinical practice. Commonly, if there is heart blood vacuity, this merely complicates liver depression and spleen vacuity. If the liver depression is secondary in importance, then one would choose a guiding formula which primarily supplements and nourishes the heart and spleen, modifying it for liver depression. If liver depression is primary, then one would modify a formula from under that pattern.

Yin vacuity, fire effulgence

Main symptoms: Heart vexation, insomnia, heart palpitations worsened in the evening or due to stress, menstruation either early or late, lumbar soreness, numb extremities, one-sided headache, tinnitus, blurred vision, distention and pain that feels as if it stretches from the lower abdomen to the chest and breasts, frequent, short urination, length of menstruation short and amount profuse, a dry mouth with scanty fluids, a red tongue with scanty, shiny, or peeled fur, and a fine, rapid, bowstring pulse

Treatment principles: Supplement the kidneys and enrich yin, regulate the liver and downbear fire

Although not stated in the Chinese title of this pattern, liver qi depression and stagnation are a part of this scenario. This is evidenced by the feeling of lower abdominal distention and pain reaching to the chest and breasts and also by the bowstring pulse.

---

[5] A soggy pulse is another of the main 28 pulse images of Chinese medicine. It refers to a pulse which is floating, fine, and forceless.

Heart & kidneys not interacting

Main symptoms: Vexation and agitation, vexatious heat in the center of the heart, restlessness, severe, continuous palpitations or racing heart, coolness of the lower limbs, great difficulty falling asleep, a red tongue with dry, yellow fur, and a fine, rapid or surging pulse

Treatment principles: Clear the heart and lead yang to move downward to its lower origin

As discussed above, the pattern of heart and kidneys not interacting is an extreme form of yin vacuity with yang heat counterflowing upward to accumulate and disturb the spirit residing in the heart.

Heart vacuity, gallbladder timidity

Main symptoms: Timidity, susceptibility to fright, fatigue, heart palpitations, shortness of breath, reduced sleep, profuse dreaming, waking in a startle or fright

Treatment principles: Supplement the qi, nourish the heart, and quiet the gallbladder

This pattern is actually fairly complex. Although the name of the pattern does not say this in so many words, there is spleen qi vacuity leading to a heart and lung qi vacuity on the one hand and an accumulation of dampness and phlegm on the other. There is also heart blood vacuity and liver depression qi stagnation. When the treatment principles say to supplement the qi, this means the heart and lung qi which is essentially derived from the spleen qi. When we say to nourish the heart, this means to nourish the heart blood. And when we say to quiet the gallbladder, this means to course the liver and rectify the qi. Although the treatment principles do not say this, one must also eliminate dampness and transform phlegm.

Phlegm heat internally harassing

Main symptoms: Insomnia, a heavy, full, stuffy, or tight feeling in the head, excessive or profuse phlegm, chest oppression,[6] aversion to food, burping and belching, acid regurgitation, possible nausea, heart vexation,[7] a bitter taste in the mouth, vertigo and dizziness, slimy, yellow tongue fur, and a slippery, rapid, possibly also bowstring pulse

Treatment principles: Transform phlegm and clear heat, harmonize the center and quiet the spirit

As in the pattern above, the name of this pattern and its treatment principles do not completely describe the mechanisms causing these signs and symptoms. Harmonizing the center means to harmonize and regulate the upbearing and downbearing of the qi mechanism. The nausea, belching, and acid regurgitation all evidence that there is upward counterflow. Most commonly, this upward counterflow is due to liver depression qi stagnation resulting in counterflow. If qi backs up and accumulates, eventually it must vent itself somewhere. Since it is yang, it typically vents itself upward. In addition, extreme or enduring depression has transformed into heat or even fire.

---

[6] Chest oppression refers to a feeling of tightness and stuffiness in the chest. As a reaction to this feeling, the person will often sigh in an attempt to inhale fresh air and exhale the pent-up stale air.

[7] Heart vexation refers to a irritating, possibly dry, hot sensation in the chest in front of the heart.

Stomach disharmony

Main symptoms: Indigestion, no thought for or aversion at the thought of food, nausea, bad breath, thick, slimy tongue fur, and a slippery pulse

Treatment principles: Downbear the stomach and disperse food

This pattern may be of recent onset due to a single bout of over-eating and drinking. In that case, it may be seen as a simple, discrete pattern as described above. However, this pattern may also complicate other patterns associated with either liver depression or phlegm. This is because the liver's control over coursing and discharging is intimately connected with the process of digestion and the downbearing of the turbid by the stomach. In addition, if there is liver depression qi stagnation and spleen vacuity giving rise to the accumulation of dampness and phlegm, it is even more likely that upbearing and downbearing have become disharmonious. This means that often symptoms of food stagnating in the stomach, such as bad breath, nausea, indigestion, thick, slimy tongue fur, and a slippery pulse, merely complicate other patterns. In that case, the treatment principles for those other patterns are amended by the addition of the principles of downbearing the stomach and dispersing food or abducting stagnation. One might also simply say to harmonize the stomach which means to downbear the stomach. If the stomach qi downbears correctly, stagnant food will automatically be dispersed and abducted or led downward to the intestines.

Blood stasis

Main symptoms: Premenstrual or menstrual lower abdominal pain which is either severe or is fixed in location and sharp or piercing in nature, varicose veins, chronic hemorrhoids, various types of lower abdominal lumps and masses, such as endometriosis, ovarian cysts, and uterine fibroids, lumps in the breast, sharp,

56

piercing pain anywhere in the body which is fixed in location and which tends to be worse in the evenings and night, a dark, dusky facial complexion or a tendency to brown spots on the skin, such as so-called age or liver spots, a purplish tongue or a tongue with static spots or static macules (*i.e.*, black and blue patches), dark, engorged, twisted and prominent veins under the tongue, and a bowstring, fine, choppy pulse[8]

Treatment principles: Quicken the blood and transform or dispel stasis

This pattern is rarely encountered as the sole pattern accounting for a person's insomnia. Therefore, most clinical manuals do not even list it. However, blood stasis does commonly complicate many people's insomnia, especially insomnia in women and in the elderly. In cases complicated by insomnia, the treatment principles for blood stasis are then added to the other treatment principles and the treatment for blood stasis is then added to other treatments for other patterns.

The real deal

Although textbook discriminations such as the one above make it seem like all the practitioner has to do is match up their patient's symptoms with one of the aforementioned patterns and then prescribe the recommended guiding formula, in actual clinical practice, one usually encounters combinations of the above discrete patterns and their related disease mechanisms or progressions. For instance, liver depression transforming heat may be complicated by spleen qi and heart blood vacuity. This, in turn may also be complicated by phlegm or blood stasis. Likewise,

---

[8] A choppy pulse means a pulse whose beat is not very regular. Although this pulse does not actually contain skipped beats, its beats tend to speed up and slow down. In addition, the force of each beat as it hits the fingertips may be variable, some beats being noticeably stronger than others.

yin vacuity with fire effulgence may be complicated by liver depression and qi vacuity, liver depression and blood stasis, or liver depression and phlegm.

In my experience as a clinician, the liver plays a central role in most people's insomnia. Because insomnia is such a stressful and frustrating experience, if liver depression qi stagnation did not originally cause a person's insomnia, they cannot have insomnia for too long before the experience of insomnia itself causes liver depression qi stagnation. As the reader can see, four out of the eight patterns of insomnia do always include liver depression as part of their inherent mechanisms, while the remaining four are all often complicated by liver depression based on Chinese medical theories pertaining to the interrelationships between the qi and blood and viscera and bowels. Therefore, attention to and remedy of the causes and mechanisms of liver depression qi stagnation are almost always useful when dealing with insomnia.

How This System Works in Real-life

Using all the above information on the theory of Chinese medicine and the patterns and their mechanisms of insomnia, let's see how a Chinese doctor makes this system work in real-life.

Jocelyne's case

Take Jocelyne, for instance, whom I introduced at the beginning of this book. She has been having insomnia for several weeks. Specifically, Jocelyne has been having trouble getting to sleep. Once she gets to sleep, she has many disturbing dreams and often finds herself waking in a panic. Jocelyne is 38 years old. She is somewhat overweight but has a very strong, fairly solid body. When Jocelyne gets under stress, she often feels a lump in the back of her throat as if there was something there which she could neither swallow down nor spit up. She describes this as "postnasal drip" and says that she typically does hack up some white phlegm every morning when taking her shower. Jocelyne also says that she often has headaches which feel like a tight band around her head. Her chest feels stuffy and tight and she often sighs. When she really gets stressed, she feels some pain in her left chest or ribs. That scares her and she worries about having a heart attack. This fear of heart attack is worsened by the presence of heart palpitations when she gets nervous or stressed.

Lately, Jocelyne has noticed that she is frequently getting red, painful sores on the tip of her tongue and is waking with a bitter taste in her mouth. Also when she wakes, her mouth is very dry and she is very thirsty. Jocelyne's insomnia gets worse before her menstruation, at which time she also has sore, swollen breasts, lower abdominal distention, and a tendency to constipation which turns to diarrhea on the first day of her period. She has had moderately painful cramps on the first day of her period for years, "Doesn't everyone?" In general, Jocelyne says she is and has been depressed for a long time. When I ask her what depression means to her, she says it is a combination of feeling fatigued and irritable at the same time. When I ask her to stick out her tongue, it is somewhat redder than normal, especially on its tip and edges, and it has slightly dry, yellow, somewhat slimy fur or coating. Her pulse is bowstring, slippery, and rapid, but also bowstring and soggy just over the wrist bone on her right hand.

How a Chinese doctor analyzes Jocelyne's symptoms

In Chinese medicine, difficulty falling asleep initially is usually due more to hyperactivity of yang than vacuity of yin or blood. The facts that Jocelyne is slightly overweight, has headaches like a tight band around her head, and has excessive phlegm all suggest that phlegm dampness is playing a part in her total pattern or picture. The feeling of phegm in the back of her throat is called plum pit qi in Chinese medicine and is an indication of upwardly counterflowing phlegm lodged in the throat due to liver depression qi stagnation in turn due to stress. This is confirmed by Jocelyne's premenstrual breast distention and pain, chest and rib pain, premenstrual and menstrual lower abdominal pain, constipation before the onset of her menses, irritability, and bowstring pulse, all of which when taken together in Chinese medicine are seen as emblems of liver depression qi stagnation. The bitter taste in her mouth in the morning shows that enduring or extreme depression has transformed into heat. This is confirmed by the red tongue tip and edges, the rapid pulse, the yellow tongue fur, and the sores on the tip of the tongue, all of which indicate heat. The slimy fur and the slippery pulse indicate phlegm. The loose stools at the onset of the menses, the fatigue, and the soggy pulse in the pulse position associated with the spleen all indicate that Jocelyne's phlegm is, in part, due to spleen qi vacuity not moving and transforming fluids which then gather and accumulate, first transforming into dampness and then congealing into phlegm.

Therefore, the Chinese doctor knows that there is phlegm fire due to a combination of liver depression transforming heat and spleen vacuity engendering dampness and then phlegm. The insomnia is thus due to phlegm confounding the portals of the heart at the same time as fire harassing the heart spirit. This leads to insomnia, heart palpitations, and disturbing, profuse dreams.

How a Chinese doctor treats Jocelyne's insomnia

Once a Chinese doctor knows the patient's pattern discrimination, the next step is to formulate the treatment principles necessary to rebalance the imbalance implied by this pattern discrimination. If the Chinese doctor listed phlegm fire or heat as the main pattern, then the treatment principles are to transform phlegm and downbear fire or clear heat. If the Chinese doctor said that, secondarily, there is liver depression transforming heat, then they would add the principles of coursing the liver and resolving depression. Further, if phlegm is due to spleen vacuity not moving and transforming body fluids, then one should also fortify the spleen and supplement the qi.

Once the Chinese doctor has stated the treatment principles, then they know that anything which works to accomplish these principles will be good for the patient. Using these principles, the Chinese doctor can now select various acupuncture points which achieve these effects. They can prescribe Chinese herbal medicinals which embody these principles. They can make recommendations about what to eat and not eat based on these principles. They can make recommendations on lifestyle changes. And, in short, they can advise the patient on *any and every aspect of their life*, judging whether something either aids the accomplishment of these principles or works against it.

In Chinese medicine, the internal administration of Chinese "herbal" medicinals is the main modality.[9] So let's look at how a Chinese doctor crafts a prescription for Jocelyne. Because the first treatment principle stated for Jocelyne is to transform phlegm, the Chinese doctor knows that he or she should select their guiding formula from the phlegm-transforming category of formulas. Depending on the textbook, there are 22-28 main categories of formulas in Chinese medicine, each category correlated to a main treatment principle. The category of phlegm-transforming formulas is subdivided into formulas which transform and clear phlegm heat and those which transform and warm phlegm cold. Since Jocelyne's case has to do with phlegm fire, we need to pick a formula from those which transform phlegm and clear heat or fire.

Under this category of formulas, there are some formulas which mainly treat respiratory tract problems, such as bronchitis, pneumonia, asthma, and whooping cough. Since Jocelyne's main complaint is insomnia, we must look for a formula which is empirically known through clinical experience to treat insomnia. Very quickly the list narrows down to one very famous formula, *Huang Lian Wen Dan Tang* (Coptis Warm the Gallbladder Decoction). This formula is for the treatment of insomnia, excessive fright, and heart palpitations due to a combination of

---

[9] I've put the word herbal in quotation marks since Chinese medicine is not entirely herbal. Herbs are medicinals made from parts of plants, their roots, bark, stems, leaves, flowers, etc. Chinese medicinals are mostly herbal in nature. However, a percentage of Chinese medicinals also come from the animal and mineral realms. Thus not all Chinese medicinals are, strictly speaking, herbs.

liver depression transforming heat and phlegm harassing the heart. Since liver depression is already a part of this formula's rationale, we may not need to add anything more for the liver depression qi stagnation we have identified at work in Jocelyne. However, this formula does not include anything for fortifying the spleen and supplementing the qi. Therefore, we will have to add some ingredients for these purposes.

Hence the final formula composed by the Chinese doctor will be called *Huang Lian Wen Dan Tang Jia Wei* (Coptis Warm the Gallbladder Decoction with Added Flavors [*i.e.*, Ingredients]). This formula is comprised of:

Radix Coodnopsitis Pilosulae (*Dang Shen*)
Rhizoma Coptidis Chinensis (*Huang Lian*)
Caulis Bambusae In Taeniis (*Zhu Ru*)
Rhizoma Pinelliae Teranatae (*Ban Xia*)
Sclerotium Poriae Cocos (*Fu Ling*)
Pericarpium Citri Reticulatae (*Chen Pi*)
Fructus Immaturus Citri Aurantii (*Zhi Shi*)
Radix Glycyrrhizae (*Gan Cao*)
uncooked Rhizoma Zingiberis (*Sheng Jiang*)

Radix Codonopsitis fortifies the spleen and supplements the qi. It is not part of the standard prescription but is added in order to take care of and embody those treatment principles having to do with Jocelyne's spleen qi vacuity which is connected with her engenderment of phlegm and dampness. Rhizoma Coptidis is bitter and cold and clears heat from the liver, stomach, and heart. Therefore, it is very good for eliminating depressive heat affecting the heart but originating in the liver. Caulis Bambusae also clears depressive heat in the liver at the same time as it elimates vexation, that hot sense of irritability in the chest. Further, Caulis Bambusae downbears the stomach, thus downbearing upwardly counterflowing depressive heat. Rhizoma Pinelliae likewise harmonizes or downbears the stomach. It also transforms phlegm and eliminates dampness via the spleen's movement and transformation. Pinellia is aided in this by Sclerotium Poriae which fortifies the spleen and eliminates dampness via urination. Poria also supplements the heart qi and quiets the spirit. Pericarpium Citri is aged Orange or Tangerine Peel. It helps Pinellia transform phlegm dampness at the same time as it helps Bambusa regulate the downbearing of qi. Likewise Fructus Immaturus Citri, immature Aurantium fruit, even more strongly rectifies and regulates the qi. Together, these last two ingredients can help eliminate premenstrual breast distention due to liver depression qi stagnation. Radix Glycyrrhizae or Licorice supplements the spleen and heart. It also helps harmonize all the other ingredients in the formula and prevents them from having unwanted side effects. While uncooked Rhizoma Zingiberis or Ginger helps eliminate dampness and transform phlegm at the same time as it harmonizes the stomach and promotes the movement of qi.

Hence one can see that the ingredients in this formula very precisely and specifically embody and carry out the treatment principles we have said were necessary for rebalancing Jocelyne's condition. To make this formula even more effective, the Chinese doctor will also rarely prescribe this formula in its textbook form above. Rather, we will modify it even further by taking out one or more ingredients and adding others as necessary in order to tailor it to the individual patient's exact configuration of signs and symptoms. Since Jocelyne experiences premenstrual and menstrual abdominal cramping, during her premenstruum, I would first add Rhizoma Cyperi Rotundi (*Xiang Fu*) and Rhizoma Corydalis Yanhusuo (*Yan Hu Suo*) to further move the qi and stop pain. To further eliminate the premenstrual breast distention and pain at the same time as quieting the spirit and improving the sleep, I would add Semen Citri Reticulatae (*Ju He*) and Cortex Albizziae Julibrissin (*He Huan Pi*). For the loose stools at the onset of the period, I might add Rhizoma Atractylodis Macrocephalae (*Bai Zhu*) to fortify the spleen even more and dry dampness. However, since depressive heat has damaged fluids somewhat, as evidenced by the thirst and dry mouth on waking in the morning, I would probably add Tuber Ophiopogonis Japonici (*Mai Dong*). This ingredient would not only enrich stomach fluids but also clear heat from the heart at the same time as transforming phlegm.

Usually, a formula such as this when used to treat insomnia would be taken two to three times each day. The herbs would be soaked in water and then boiled into a very strong "tea" for 30-45 minutes. Since insomnia is Jocelyne's major complaint, I would probably have her begin taking this "tea" at noon, with the third or last dose being taken a half hour before bed in order to insure its effect being strong and targeted for the second half of the day. Each week, I would check with Jocelyne to see how she was doing and if I needed to make any modifications to her formula. Remember, the Chinese doctor wants to heal without causing *any* side effects. If the formula does cause any unwanted effects, then it is my job to add and subtract ingredients until it achieves a perfect result with no unwanted effects.

The ingredients in this formula may also be taken as a dried, powdered extract. Such extracts are manufactured by several Taiwanese and Japanese companies. Although such extracts are not, in my experience, as powerful as the freshly decocted "teas", they are easier to take. Many standard formulas also come as ready-made pills. However, these cannot be modified. If their ingredients match the individual patient's requirements, then they are fine. If the formula needs modifications, then teas or powders whose individual ingredients can be added and subtracted are necessary.

In exactly the same way, the Chinese doctor could create an individualized acupuncture treatment plan and would certainly create an accompanying dietary and lifestyle plan. However, we will discuss each of these in their own chapter. In a woman

65

Jocelyne's age with her Chinese pattern discrimination, either Chinese herbal medicine alone, acupuncture alone, or a combination of the two supported by the proper diet and lifestyle will usually eliminate or at the very least drastically diminish her insomnia within three to five days. Often results will be apparent the first night after taking the herbs for a full day. However, the reader should understand that such Chinese medicinals are not like sedatives. One cannot simply take them at bedtime and expect to get a sound night's sleep. Chinese medicinals such as these act to restore balance and harmony to the yin and yang of the body. Therefore, they do not usually provide immediate symptomatic relief to insomnia in the same way as taking a Valium. Conversely, they also do not cause any drowsiness or grogginess the next day.

Chinese Herbal Medicine & Insomnia

As we have seen from Jocelyne's case above, there is no Chinese "insomnia herb" or even an "insomnia formula" which will work for all sufferers of insomnia. Chinese medicinals are individually prescribed based on a person's pattern discrimination, not on a disease diagnosis like insomnia. Patients often come to me and say, "My friend told me that *Tian Wang Bu Xin Dan* (Heavenly Emperor Supplement the Heart Elixir, a common Chinese over-the-counter medication) is good for insomnia. But I tried it and it didn't work." This is because *Tian Wang Bu Xin Dan* is meant to treat a *specific pattern* of insomnia, not insomnia per se. If you exhibit that pattern, then this formula will work. If you do not have signs and symptoms of this pattern, it won't.

In addition, because most people's insomnia is a combination of different Chinese patterns and disease mechanisms, professional Chinese medicine never treats insomnia with herbal "singles." In herbalism, singles mean the prescription of a single herb all by itself. Chinese herbal medicine is based on rebalancing patterns, and patterns in real-life patients almost always have more than a single element. Therefore, Chinese doctors almost always prescribe herbs in multi-ingredient formulas. Such formulas may have anywhere from six to eighteen or more ingredients. When a Chinese doctor reads a prescription by another Chinese doctor, they can tell you not only what the patient's pattern discrimination is but also their probable signs and symptoms. In other words, the Chinese doctor does not just combine several medicinals which are all reputed to be "good for insomnia." Rather, they carefully craft a formula whose ingredients are meant to rebalance every aspect of the patient's body-mind.

Getting your own individualized prescription

Since, in China, it takes not less than four years of full-time college education to learn how to do a professional Chinese pattern discrimination and then write an herbal formula based on that pattern discrimination, most laypeople cannot realistically write their own Chinese herbal prescriptions. It should also be remembered that Chinese herbs are not effective and safe because they are either Chinese or herbal. In fact, approximately 20% of the common Chinese materia medica did not originate in Chinese, and not all Chinese herbs are completely safe. They are only safe when prescribed according to a correct pattern discrimination, in the right dose, and for the right amount of time. After all, if an herb is strong enough to heal an imbalance, it is also strong enough to create an imbalance if overdosed or misprescribed. Therefore, I strongly recommend persons who wish to experience the many benefits of Chinese herbal medicine to see a qualified professional practitioner who can do a professional pattern discrimination and write you an individualized prescription. Towards the end of this book, I will give the reader suggestions on how to find a qualified professional Chinese medical practitioner near you.

Experimenting with Chinese patent medicines

In reality, qualified professional practitioners of Chinese medicine are not yet found in every North American community. In addition, some people may want to try to heal their insomnia as much on their own as possible. More and more health food stores are stocking a variety of ready-made Chinese formulas in pill and powder form. These ready-made, over-the-counter Chinese

68

medicines are often referred to as Chinese patent medicines. Although my best recommendation is for readers to seek Chinese herbal treatment from professional practitioners, below are some suggestions of how one might experiment with Chinese patent medicines to treat insomnia.

In chapter 5, I have given the signs and symptoms of the eight key or basic patterns associated with most people's insomnia. These are:

1. Liver depression qi stagnation
2. Liver depression transforming into heat
3. Yin vacuity, fire effulgence
4. Heart & kidneys not interacting
5. Heart-spleen dual vacuity
6. Heart vacuity, gallbladder timidity
7. Stomach disharmony
8. Blood stasis

If the reader can identify their main pattern from chapter 5, then there are some Chinese patent remedies that they might consider trying.

Xiao Yao Wan (also spelled *Hsiao Yao Wan*)

Xiao Yao Wan is one of the most common Chinese herbal formulas prescribed. Its Chinese name has been translated as Free & Easy Pills, Rambling Pills, Relaxed Wanderer Pills, and several other versions of this same idea of promoting a freer and smoother, more relaxed flow. As a patent medicine, this formula comes as pills, and there are both Chinese-made and American-made versions of this formula available over-the-counter in the North American marketplace.[10]

The ingredients in this formula are:

Radix Bupleuri (*Chai Hu*)
Radix Angelicae Sinensis (*Dang Gui*)
Radix Albus Paeoniae Lactiflorae (*Bai Shao*)
Rhizoma Atractylodis Macrocephalae (*Bai Zhu*)
Sclerotium Poriae Cocos (*Fu Ling*)
mix-fried Radx Glycyrrhizae (*Gan Cao*)
Herba Menthae Haplocalycis (*Bo He*)
uncooked Rhizoma Zingiberis (*Sheng Jiang*)

This formula treats the pattern of liver depression qi stagnation complicated by blood vacuity and spleen weakness with possible dampness as well. Bupleurum courses the liver and rectifies the qi. It is aided in this by Herba Menthae Haplocalycis or Peppermint. Dang Gui and Radix Albus Paeoniae Lactilforae or White Peony nourish the blood and soften and harmonize the liver. Rhizoma Atractylodis Macrocephalae or Atractylodes and Sclerotium Poriae Cocos or Poria fortify the spleen and eliminate dampness. Mix-fried Licorice aid these two in fortifying the spleen and supplementing the liver, while uncooked Ginger aids in both promoting and regulating the qi flow and eliminating dampness.

When insomnia presents with the signs and symptoms of liver depression, spleen qi vacuity, and an element of blood vacuity, one can try taking this formula. However, after taking these pills at the dose recommended on the package, if one notices any side effects, then stop immediately and seek a professional consultation. Such side effects from this formula might include

---

[10] When marketed as a dried, powdered extract, this formula is sold under the name of Bupleurum & Tang-kuei Formula.

nervousness, irritability, a dry mouth and increased thirst, and red, dry eyes. Such side effects show that this formula, at least without modification, is not right for you. Although it may be doing you some good, it is also causing some harm. Remember, Chinese medicine is meant to cure without side effects, and as long as the prescription matches one's pattern there will not be any.

Dan Zhi Xiao Yao Wan

Dan Zhi Xiao Yao Wan or Moutan & Gardenia Rambling Pills is a modification of the above formula which also comes as a patent medicine in the form of pills.[11] It is meant to treat the pattern of liver depression transforming into heat with spleen vacuity and possible blood vacuity and/or dampness. The ingredients in this formula are the same as above except that two other herbs are added:

Cortex Radicis Moutan (*Dan Pi*)
Fructus Gardeniae Jasminoidis (*Shan Zhi Zi*)

These two ingredients clear heat and resolve depression. In addition, Cortex Radicis Moutan or Moutan quickens the blood and dispels stasis and is good at clearing heat specifically from the blood. Some Chinese doctors say to take out uncooked Ginger and Mint, while others leave these two ingredients in.

Basically, the signs and symptoms of the pattern for which this formula is designed are the same as those for *Xiao Yao San* above plus signs and symptoms of depressive heat. These might include a reddish tongue with slightly yellow fur, a bowstring and rapid pulse, a bitter taste in the mouth, and increased irritability.

---

[11] When marketed as a dried, powdered extract, this formula is called Bupleurum & Peony Formula.

71

Tabellae *Suan Zao Ren Tang*

This is a tableted version of the formula, *Suan Zao Ren Tang* (Zizyphus Seed Decoction).[12] It treats insomnia and mental unrest due to liver blood vacuity. It can, therefore, be combined with *Xiao Yao Wan* when liver blood vacuity is more severe and manifests primarily as insomnia. Its ingredients are:

Semen Zizyphi Spinosae (*Suan Zao Ren*)
Sclerotium Poriae Cocos (*Fu Ling*)
Radix Ligustici Wallichii (*Chuan Xiong*)
Rhizoma Anemarrhenae Aspheloidis (*Zhi Mu*)
mix-fried Radix Glycyrrhizae (*Gan Cao*)

Gui Pi Wan (also spelled *Kuei Pi Wan*)

Gui means to return or restore, *pi* means the spleen, and *wan* means pills. Therefore, the name of these pills means Restore the Spleen Pills.[13] However, these pills not only supplement the spleen qi but also nourish heart blood and calm the heart spirit. They are the textbook guiding formula for the pattern of heart-spleen dual vacuity. In this case, there are symptoms of spleen qi vacuity, such as fatigue, poor appetite, and cold hands and feet plus symptoms of heart blood vacuity, such as a pale tongue, heart palpitations, and insomnia. This formula is also the standard one for treating heavy or abnormal bleeding due to the spleen not containing and restraining the blood within its vessels. Therefore, this patent medicine can be combined with *Xiao Yao San* when there is liver depression qi stagnation complicated by heart blood and spleen qi vacuity. Its ingredients are:

---

[12] When sold as a dried, powdered extract, this formula is called Zizyphus Combination.

[13] When sold as a dried, powdered extract, this formula is called Ginseng & Longan Combination.

Radix Astragali Membranacei (*Huang Qi*)
Radix Codonopsitis Pilosulae (*Dang Shen*)
Rhizoma Atractylodis Macrocephalae (*Bai Zhu*)
Sclerotium Parardicis Poriae Cocos (*Fu Shen*)
mix-fried Radix Glycyrrhizae (*Gan Cao*)
Radix Angelicae Sinensis (*Dang Gui*)
Semen Zizyphi Spinosae (*Suan Zao Ren*)
Arillus Euphoriae Longanae (*Long Yan Rou*)
Radix Polygalae Tenuifoliae (*Yuan Zhi*)
Radix Auklandiae Lappae (*Mu Xiang*)

Tian Wang Bu Xin Dan

The name of this formula translates as Heavenly Emperor's Supplement the Heart Elixir.[14] This formula comes as a Chinese patent medicine in pill form. It treats insomnia, restlessness, fatigue, and heart palpitations due to yin, blood, and qi vacuity, with an emphasis on heart yin and liver blood vacuity. Its ingredients include:

uncooked Radix Rehmanniae (*Sheng Di*)
Radix Scrophulariae Ninpoensis (*Xuan Shen*)
Fructus Schisandrae Chinensis (*Wu Wei Zi*)
Tuber Asparagi Cochinensis (*Tian Men Dong*)
Tuber Ophiopogonis Japonici (*Mai Men Dong*)
Radix Angelicae Sinensis (*Dang Gui*)
Semen Biotae Orientalis (*Bai Zi Ren*)
Semen Zizyphi Spinosae (*Suan Zao Ren*)
Radix Salviae Miltiorrhizae (*Dan Shen*)
Radix Polygalae Tenuifoliae (*Yuan Zhi*)
Sclerotium Poriae Cocos (*Fu Ling*)
Radix Codonopositis Pilosulae (*Dang Shen*)

---

[14] When marketed as a desiccated, powdered extract, this formula is sold under the name Ginseng & Zizyphus Formula.

Bai Zi Yang Xin Wan (also spelled *Pai Tsu Yang Xin Wan*)

The name of this formula translates as Biotae Nourish the Heart Pills. Another commonly used over-the-counter Chinese patent pill for insomnia, this formula is for heart yin and liver blood vacuity complicated by an element of phlegm obstruction. Its ingredients include:

Semen Biotae Orientalis (*Bai Zi Ren*)
Fructus Lycii Chinensis (*Gou Qi Zi*)
Radix Scrophulariae Ningpoensis (*Xuan Shen*)
uncooked Radix Rehmanniae (*Sheng Di*)
Tuber Ophiopogonis Japonici (*Mai Men Dong*)
Radix Angelicae Sinensis (*Dang Gui*)
Sclerotium Poriae Cocos (*Fu Ling*)
Rhizoma Acori Graminei (*Shi Chang Pu*)
Radix Glycyrrhizae (*Gan Cao*)

Bu Nao Wan

Similar to the above two formulas, Supplement the Brain Pills are another popular Chinese patent pill for insomnia, restlessness, heart palpitations, and poor memory. Their name is popularly mis- or overtranslated as Cerebral Tonic Pills. The pattern they are designed to remedy is a yin and yang vacuity, with emphasis on the blood and yin vacuity, plus internal stirring of wind due to yin vacuity with upward counterflow confounding or obstructing the portals of the heart. In this case, there is most likely also an element of liver depression which this formula does address.

We have not previously mentioned internal stirring of wind as a cause or type of insomnia. Internal stirring of wind here refers to upwardly counterflowing yang qi which is moving extremely frenetically or recklessly. It is indicated by dizziness and vertigo, tremors and spasms, and a quivering tongue. Besides insomnia, other conditions associated with this group of disease mechanisms are epilepsy, apoplexy, mania, and seizures. Although there are no particular signs of heat or fire, the symptoms of ascendant liver wind are pronounced. The ingredients in this formula are:

Fructus Schisandrae Chinensis (*Wu Wei Zi*)
Semen Zizyphi Spinosae (*Suan Zao Ren*)
Radix Angelicae Sinensis (*Dang Gui*)
Fructus Lycii Chinensis (*Gou Qi Zi*)
Herba Cistanchis Deserticolae (*Rou Cong Rong*)
Semen Juglandis Regiae (*Hu Tao Ren*)
Semen Biotae Orientalis (*Bai Zi Ren*)
Rhizoma Acori Graminaei (*Shi Chang Pu*)
Rhizoma Arisaematis (*Nan Xing*)
Radix Gastrodiae Elatae (*Tian Ma*)
Succinum (*Hu Po*)
Dens Draconis (*Long Chi*)
Radix Polygalae Tenuifoliae (*Yuan Zhi*)

An Shen Bu Xin Wan (also spelled *An Shen Pu Shin Wan*)

An shen means to quiet the spirit. *Bu xin* means to supplement the heart. Therefore, the Chinese name for these pills means Quiet the Spirit & Supplement the Heart Pills. This is yet another Chinese patent pill designed to treat insomnia, dizziness, restlessness, profuse dreaming which disturbs the sleep, and heart palpitations due to yin and blood vacuity. Its ingredients also take into account an element of liver depression qi stagnation and an element of phlegm obstruction. In addition, because the ingredient with the largest dose in this formula is Mother of Pearl Powder, this formula helps to downbear upwardly counterflowing yang qi and quiet the spirit quite strongly. All its ingredients are:

Concha Maragaritiferae (*Zhen Zhu Mu*)
Radix Polygoni Multiflori (*He Shou Wu*)
Fructus Ligustri Lucidi (*Nu Zhen Zi*)
Herba Ecliptae Prostratae (*Han Lian Cao*)

Semen Cuscutae Chinensis (*Tu Si Zi*)
Fructus Schisandrae Chinensis (*Wu Wei Zi*)
Radix Salviae Miltiorrhizae (*Dan Shen*)
Cortex Albizziae Julibrissin (*He Huan Pi*)
Rhizoma Acori Graminei (*Shi Chang Pu*)

Zhu Sha An Shen Wan

The Chinese name of this formula means Cinnabar Quiet the Spirit Pills. This is mistranslated as Cinnabar Sedative Pills on the box. It is for heart and kidneys not interacting, or, in other words, fairly pronounced yin vacuity with upward counterflow of yang or even fire in the heart. Its ingredients are:

Radix Angelicae Sinensis (*Dang Gui*)
uncooked Radix Rehmanniae (*Sheng Di*)
Rhizoma Coptidis Chinensis (*Huang Lian*)
Radix Glycyrrhize (*Gan Cao*)
Cinnabar (*Zhu Sha*)

This pill should only be taken for a very short period of time in order to calm intense insomnia and restlessness due to the heart and kidneys not interacting. As soon as the person is able to sleep at all, one should switch to a more moderate, safer pill. Cinnabar is a mercuric compound. It has been used for millenia in China as a spirit-quieting medicinal. However, mercury is toxic if ingested for any length of time. Mercury's toxic effect is cumulative. Therefore, one should be sure not to use this formula for more than a few days. By more moderate formula, I mean a formula which pays more attention to enriching yin and nourishing the blood and less attention to clearing heat and quieting the spirit.

An altogether safer way of treating this pattern of insomnia is with an individually prescribed formula made from bulk dispensed Chinese medicinals. In that case, there is no need to use such a toxic medicinal as Cinnabar, even for this relatively extreme pattern. Therefore, if one thinks that their pattern of insomnia is the heart and kidneys not interacting pattern described above, my best advice is to seek out a professional practitioner of Chinese medicine and not try to treat this yourself with Chinese patent pills.

Jiang Ya Wan (also spelled Chiang Ya Wan)

Jiang ya means to decrease pressure as in high blood pressure. *Wan* as we've seen before means pills. These pills are usually used to treat high blood pressure due to kidney vacuity and liver effulgence. The reader should remember that actually Chinese medicine treats patterns of imbalance, not diseases such as high blood pressure. Also remember the saying, "Different diseases, same treatment." Therefore, these pills can be used to treat insomnia due to an upward flaring of liver fire or wind in turn due to loss of control by kidney yin below. Since this formula already includes medicinals for treating the liver, it would not be combined with *Xiao Yao Wan* above but used by itself. Its ingredients are:

Semen Leonuri Heterophyli (*Chong Wei Zi*)
Rhizoma Coptidis Chinensis (*Huang Lian*)
Cornu Antelopis Saiga-tatarici (*Ling Yang Jiao*)
Spica Prunellae Vulgaris (*Xia Ku Cao*)
Ramulus Uncariae Cum Uncis (*Gou Teng*)
Radix Gastrodiae Elatae (*Tian Ma*)
Succinum (*Hu Po*)
Radix Angelicae Sinensis (*Dang Gui*)
Radix Ligustici Wallichii (*Chuan Xiong*)
uncooked Radix Rehmanniae (*Sheng Di*)
Gelatinum Corii Asini (*E Jiao*)
Cortex Radicis Moutan (*Dan Pi*)
Radix Achyranthis Bidentatae (*Niu Xi*)
Lignum Aquilariae Agallochae (*Chen Xiang*)
Radix Et Rhizoma Rhei (*Da Huang*)

Because this formula contains Radix Et Rhizoma Rhei or Rhubarb which is a strong purgative, it should not be taken if one has diarrhea or loose stools. If this formula causes diarrhea, its use should be discontinued.

Kang Ning Wan

Kang means health and *ning* means tranquil. Therefore, *Kang Ning Wan* means Healthy Tranquility Pills. They are sold under the mis- or overtranslation of Curing Pills. These pills are one of several commonly found Chinese over-the-counter pills for the treatment of indigestion due to overeating and food stagnation. When insomnia is due to overeating and overdrinking, one can take these pills before going to bed. Their ingredients are:

Semen Coicis Lachryma-jobi (*Yi Yi Ren*)
Cortex Magnoliae Officinalis (*Hou Po*)
Rhizoma Atractylodis (*Cang Zhu*)
Herba Agastachis Seu Pogostemi (*Huo Xiang*)
Radix Puerariae (*Ge Gen*)
Radix Angelicae Dahuricae (*Bai Zhi*)
Radix Auklandiae Lappae (*Mu Xiang*)
Massa Medica Fermentata (*Shen Qu*)
Radix Trichosanthis Kirlowii (*Tian Hua Fen*)
Fructus Germinatus Oryzae Sativae (*Gu Ya*)
Sclerotium Poriae Cocos (*Fu Ling*)
Rhizoma Gastrodiae Elatae (*Tian Ma*)
Flos Chrysanthemi Morifolii (*Ju Hua*)
Herba Menthae Haplocalycis (*Bo He*)
Pericarpium Citri Reticulatae (*Chen Pi*)

When food stagnation complicates liver depression qi stagnation or liver depression transforming heat, these pills may be combined with *Xiao Yao San* or *Dan Zhi Xiao Yao San* discussed above.

Er Chen Wan

Er Chen Wan means Two Aged (Ingredients) Pills.[15] This is because, two of its main ingredients are aged before using. This formula is used to transform phlegm and eliminate dampness. It can be added to Xiao Yao Wan if there is liver depression with spleen vacuity and more pronounced phlegm and dampness. If there is liver depression transforming heat giving rise to phlegm heat, it can be combined with Dan Zhi Xiao Yao Wan. Its ingredients include:

Rhizoma Pinelliae Ternatae (Ban Xia)
Sclerotium Poriae Cocos (Fu Ling)
mix-fried Radix Glycyrrhizae (Gan Cao)
Pericarpium Citri Reticulatae (Chen Pi)
uncooked Rhizoma Zingiberis (Sheng Jiang)

Tong Jing Wan (also spelled To Jing Wan)

The name of these pills means Painful Menstruation Pills. They are not an "insomnia pill" per se. However, insomnia is often complicated by blood stasis in women and the elderly. Therefore, this pill can be taken along with other appropriate formulas when blood stasis is an important factor in someone's insomnia. Its ingredients are:

Tuber Curcumae (Yu Jin)
Rhizoma Sparganii (San Leng)
Radix Rubrus Paeoniae Lactiflorae (Chi Shao)
Radix Angelicae Sinensis (Dang Gui)
Radix Ligustici Wallichii (Chuan Xiong)
Radix Salviae Miltiorrhizae (Dan Shen)
Flos Carthami Tinctorii (Hong Hua)

---

[15] When sold as a dried, powdered extract, this formula is called Citrus & Pinellia Combination.

The above Chinese patent medicines only give a suggestion of how one or several over-the-counter Chinese ready-made preparations may be used to treat insomnia. As a professional practitioner of Chinese medicine, I prefer to see people receive a professional diagnosis and an individually tailored prescription. However, as long as one is careful to try to match up their pattern with the right formula and not to exceed the recommended dosages, one can try treating their insomnia with one or more of these remedies. If it works, great! These patent medicines are usually quite cheap. If this approach doesn't work after one week or there are *any side effects*, one should stop and see a professional practitioner.

Six guideposts for assessing any over-the-counter medication

In general, you can tell if any medication and treatment are good for you by checking the following six guideposts.

1. Digestion
2. Elimination
3. Energy level

4. Mood
5. Appetite
6. Sleep

If a medication, be it modern Western or traditional Chinese, gets rid of your symptoms and all six of these basic areas of human health improve, then that medicine or treatment is probably OK. However, even if a treatment or medication takes away your major complaint, *if it causes deterioration in any one of these six basic parameters,* then that treatment or medication is probably not OK and is certainly not OK for long-term use. When medicines and treatments, even so-called natural, herbal medications, are prescribed based on a person's pattern of disharmony, then there is healing without side effects. According to Chinese medicine, this is the only kind of true healing.

Acupuncture & Moxibustion

When the average Westerner thinks of Chinese medicine, they probably first think of acupuncture. Certainly acupuncture is the best known of the various methods of treatment which go to make up Chinese medicine. However, in China, acupuncture is actually a secondary treatment modality. Most Chinese immediately think of "herbal" medicine when thinking of Chinese medicine.

Be that as it may, most professional practitioners of Chinese medicine in North America are licensed or otherwise registered and permitted to practice medicine as acupuncturists. Therefore, most such practitioners treat every patient with at least some acupuncture no matter if they also prescribe a Chinese herbal formula as well. While this "doubling up" of these two therapies is not always necessary to successfully treat most diseases, insomnia in general does respond very well to correctly prescribed and administered acupuncture.

What is acupuncture?

Acupuncture primarily means the insertion of extremely thin, sterilized, stainless steel needles into specific points on the body where Chinese doctors have known for centuries there are special concentrations of qi and blood. Therefore, these points are like switches or circuit breakers for regulating and balancing the flow of qi and blood over the channel and network system we described above. As we have seen, insomnia is due to a breakdown in the harmony between yin and yang in the body, and, in the human body, yin and yang ultimately mean the qi and blood. As we have also seen, there really is no insomnia if there is not also liver depression. Either liver depression is intimately connected with the mechanisms of insomnia to begin with, or due to the frustration and stress of insomnia, one subsequently develops liver depression. Liver depression means that the qi is stagnant. Because the qi is depressed and stagnant, it is not flowing when and where it should. Instead it counterflows or vents itself to areas of the body where it shouldn't be, attacking other organs and body tissues and making them dysfunctional.

Therefore, the Chinese patterns of insomnia typically include many signs and symptoms associated with lack of or erroneous, counterflow qi flow. In addition, the heart spirit is nothing other than an accumulation of qi within the heart. If there is enough qi in the heart, then there is consciousness or what Chinese medicine calls the spirit. Since acupuncture's forte is the regulation and rectification of the flow of qi, it is an especially good treatment mode for correcting insomnia. In that case, insertion of acupuncture needles at various points in the body moves stagnant qi in the liver and leads the qi to flow in its proper directions and amounts.

As a generic term, acupuncture also includes several other methods of stimulating acupuncture points, thus regulating the flow of qi in the body. The main other modality is moxibustion. This means the warming of acupuncture points mainly by burning dried, aged Oriental Mugwort on, near, or over acupuncture points. The purpose of this warming treatment are to 1) even more strongly stimulate the flow of qi and blood, 2) add warmth to areas of the body which are too cold, and 3) add yang qi to the body to supplement a yang qi deficiency. Other acupuncture modalities are to apply suction cups over points, to massage the points, to prick the points to allow a drop or two of blood to exit, to apply Chinese medicinals to the points, to apply magnets to the points, and to stimulate the points by either electricity or laser.

What is a typical acupuncture treatment for insomnia like?

In China, acupuncture treatments are given every day or every other day, three to five times per week depending on the nature and severity of the condition. In general, it is best if one can get acupuncture every day for the first couple of treatments if insomnia is really severe. Once the person is able to sleep a little better or to get to sleep at all, one can begin to space out the treatments to every other day and thence to once or twice a week. After three to four weeks, the treatments should be tapered off completely.

When the person comes for their appointment, the practitioner will ask them what their main symptoms are, will typically look at their tongue and its fur, and will feel the pulses at the radial arteries on both wrists. Then, they will ask the patient to lie down on a treatment table. Based on their Chinese pattern discrimination, the practitioner will select anywhere from one to eight or nine points to be needled.

The needles used today are ethylene oxide gas sterilized disposable needles. This means that they are used one time and then thrown away, just like a hypodermic syringe in a doctor's office. However, unlike relatively fat hypodermic needles, acupuncture needles are hardly thicker than a strand of hair. The skin over the point is disinfected with alcohol and the needle is quickly and deftly inserted somewhere typically between one quarter and a half inch. In some few cases, a needle may be inserted deeper than that, but most needles are only inserted relatively shallowly.

After the needle has broken the skin, the acupuncturist will usually manipulate the needle in various ways until he or she feels that the qi has "arrived." This refers to a subtle but very real feeling of resistance around the needle. When the qi arrives, the patient will usually feel a mild, dull soreness around the needle, a slight electrical feeling, a heavy feeling, or a numb or tingly feeling. All these mean that the needle has tapped the qi and that treatment will be effective. Once the qi has been tapped, then the practitioner may further adjust the qi flow by manipulating the needle in certain ways, may attach the needle to an electro-acupuncture machine in order to stimulate the point with very mild and gentle electricity, or they may simply leave the needle in place. Usually the needles are left in place from 10-20 minutes. After this, the needles are withdrawn and thrown away. *Thus there is absolutely no chance for infection from another patient.*

How are the points selected?

The points one's acupuncturist chooses to needle each treatment are selected on the basis of Chinese medical theory and the known clinical effects of certain points. Since there are different schools or styles of acupuncture, point selection tends to vary from practitioner to practitioner. However, let me present a fairly typical case from the point of view of the dominant style of acupuncture in the People's Republic of China.

Let's say the patient's main complaints are difficulty falling asleep, irritability, fatigue, heart palpitations on exertion, shortness of breath, and loose stools. Their tongue is very fat and pale with thin, white fur. Their tongue is so fat that one can clearly see the indentations of the teeth on the edges of the tongue. Their pulse is fine and bowstring. This person's Chinese pattern discrimination is liver depression with heart-spleen dual vacuity. This is a very commonly encountered Chinese pattern of disharmony in women with insomnia in their 30s.

The treatment principles necessary for remedying this case are to course the liver and rectify the qi, fortify the spleen and nourish the heart, and quiet the spirit. In order to accomplish these aims, the practitioner might select the following points:

Tai Chong (Liver 3)
San Yin Jiao (Spleen 6)
Zu San Li (Stomach 36)
Shen Men (Heart 7)

Nei Guan (Pericardium 6)
Shan Zhong (Conception Vessel 17)
Bai Hui (Governing Vessel 20)
Xin Shu (Bladder 15)
Pi Shu (Bladder 20)

In this case, *Tai Chong* courses the liver and resolves depression, moves and rectifies the qi. Since liver depression qi stagnation is a main disease mechanism either causing or contributing to this woman's insomnia, this is a main or ruling point in this treatment. Since this woman's easy anger or irritability stems from liver depression, this point also eliminates the source of this woman's vexation.

San Yin Jiao is chosen to further course the liver at the same time it fortifies the spleen. It does both these things because both the liver and spleen channels cross at this point. Further, this point is known to promote the nourishment and supplementation of yin blood.

Zu San Li is the most powerful point on the stomach channel. Because the stomach is yang and the spleen is yin and because the stomach and spleen share a mutually "exterior/interior" relationship, stimulating *Zu San Li* can bolster the spleen with yang qi from the stomach which usually has plenty to spare. In addition, the stomach channel traverses the chest and, therefore,

85

needling this point can regulate the qi in the chest. Since the heart gets its qi from the spleen, supplementing the spleen by way of the stomach is an acupuncture way of transferring qi from the stomach to the spleen and thence to the heart.

Shan Zhong is located at the level of the nipples on the chest bone between the breasts. It is a local point for freeing the flow of qi in the chest. It also helps calm the spirit and provides emotional relief.

Shen Men is a point on the heart channel which supplements the heart and quiets the spirit. *Nei Guan* is a point on the pericardium channel which frees the flow of qi in the liver and the chest at the same time as it quiets the spirit in the heart. These two points are routinely used for the treatment of various patterns of insomnia.

Bai Hui is a point on the governing vessel. It is located at the very crown of the head. Therefore, it is the most yang point on the body. Needling it can quiet the spirit and push yang qi back downward. It is also a very commonly used point for treating various patterns of insomnia.

Xin Shu and *Pi Shu* are both points on the back associated with the heart and spleen respectively. They directly connect with these two viscera and can supplement weakness and deficiencies in these two organs.

Therefore, this combination of nine points addresses this woman's Chinese pattern discrimination and her major complaints of insomnia, irritability, fatigue, heart palpitations, and loose stools. It remedies both the underlying disease mechanism and addresses certain key symptoms in a very direct and immediate way. Hence it provides symptomatic relief *at the same time* as it corrects the underlying mechanisms of these symptoms.

Does acupuncture hurt?

In Chinese, it is said that acupuncture is *bu tong*, painless. However, most patients will feel some mild soreness, heaviness, electrical tingling, or distention. When done well and sensitively, it should not be sharp, biting, burning, or really painful.

How quickly will I feel the result?

One of the best things about the acupuncture treatment of insomnia is that its effects are often immediate. Since many of the mechanisms of insomnia have to do with stuck qi, as soon as the qi is made to flow, the symptoms disappear. Therefore, many patients sleep better after the very first treatment.

In addition, because irritability and nervous tension are also mostly due to liver depression qi stagnation, most people will feel an immediate relief of irritability and tension while still on the table. Typically, one will feel a pronounced tranquility and relaxation within five to ten minutes of the insertion of the needles. Many patients do drop off to sleep for a few minutes while the needles are in place.

Who should get acupuncture?

As mentioned above, because most professional practitioners in the West are legally entitled to practice under various acupuncture laws, most acupuncturists will routinely do acupuncture on every patient. Since acupuncture's effects on insomnia are usually relatively immediate, this is usually a good thing for sufferers of insomnia. However, acupuncture is particularly effective for liver depression qi stagnation, liver depression transforming heat, stomach disharmony, and blood stasis patterns of insomnia.

When a person's insomnia mostly has to do with qi vacuity, blood vacuity, or yin vacuity, then acupuncture is not as effective as internally administered Chinese herbal medicinals. Although moxibustion can add yang qi to the body, acupuncture needles cannot add qi, blood, or yin to a body in short supply of these. The best acupuncture can do in these cases is to stimulate the various viscera and bowels which engender and transform the qi, blood, and yin. Chinese herbs, on the other hand, can directly introduce qi, blood, and yin into the body, thus supplementing vacuities and insufficiencies of these. In cases of insomnia, where qi, blood, and yin vacuities are pronounced, one should either use acupuncture with Chinese medicinals or rely on Chinese medicinals alone.

Ear acupuncture

Acupuncturists believe there is a map of the entire body in the ear and that by stimulating the corresponding points in the ear, one can remedy those areas and functions of the body. Therefore, many acupuncturists will not only needle points on the body at large but also select one or more points on the ear. In terms of insomnia, needling the point *Shen Men* (Spirit Gate) can have a profound effect on relaxing tension and irritability and improving sleep. Needling the ear points *Xin* (Heart) and *Nao* (Brain) can also have a useful sedative effect when treating insomnia.

The nice thing about ear acupuncture points is that one can use tiny "press needles" which are shaped like miniature thumbtacks. These are pressed into the points, covered with adhesive tape, and left in place for five to seven days. This method can provide continuous treatment between regularly scheduled office visits. Thus ear acupuncture is a nice way of extending the duration of an acupuncture treatment. In addition, these ear points can also be stimulated with small metal pellets, radish seeds, or tiny magnets, thus getting the benefits of stimulating these points without having to insert actual needles.

The Three Free Therapies

Although one can experiment cautiously with Chinese herbal medicinals, one cannot really do acupuncture on oneself. Therefore, Chinese herbal medicine and acupuncture and its related modalities mostly require the aid of a professional practitioner. However, there are three free therapies which are crucial to treating insomnia. These are diet, exercise, and deep relaxation. Only you can take care of these three factors in your health!

Diet

In Chinese medicine, the function of the spleen and stomach are likened to a pot on a stove or a still. The stomach receives the foods and liquids which then "rotten and ripen" like a mash in a fermentation vat. The spleen then cooks this mash and drives off (*i.e.,* transforms and upbears) the pure part. This pure part collects in the lungs to become the qi and in the heart to become the blood. In addition, Chinese medicine characterizes this transformation as a process of yang qi transforming yin substance. All the principles of Chinese dietary therapy, including what persons with insomnia should and should not eat, are derived from these basic "facts."

We have already seen that the spleen is the root of qi and blood engenderment and transformation. Based on this fact, a healthy, strong spleen prevents and treats insomnia in three ways. First, if the spleen is healthy and strong, it will create sufficient qi to push the blood and move body fluids. Therefore, a sufficiency of pushing or moving spleen qi helps counterbalance or control any tendency of the liver to constrict or constrain the qi flow. Thus, in Chinese medicine, a healthy spleen helps keeps the liver in check and free from depression and stagnation. Secondly, since the spleen is the root of blood production and it is yin blood which keeps yang qi in check, a healthy, strong spleen manufacturing abundant blood insures a sufficiency of heart blood to nourish and quiet the spirit. And third, since any qi, but especially blood, remaining unused at the end of the day can be converted into essence during sleep at night, a strong, healthy spleen manufacturing abundant qi and blood also helps insure the bolstering and supplementation of yin by acquired essence.

Therefore, when it comes to Chinese dietary therapy and insomnia, there are two main issues: 1) to avoid foods which damage the spleen, and 2) to eat foods which help build yin and blood.

Foods which damage the spleen

In terms of foods which damage the spleen, Chinese medicine begins with uncooked, chilled foods. If the process of digestion is likened to cooking, then cooking is nothing other than predigestion outside of the body. In Chinese medicine, it is a given that the overwhelming majority of all food should be cooked, *i.e.*, predigested. Although cooking may destroy some vital nutrients (in Chinese, qi), cooking does render the remaining nutrients much more easily assimilable. Therefore, even though some nutrients have been lost, the net absorption of nutrients is greater with cooked foods than raw. Further, eating raw foods makes the spleen work harder and thus wears the spleen out more quickly. If one's spleen is very robust, eating uncooked, raw foods may not be so damaging, but we have already seen that many women's spleens are already weak because of their monthly menses

THE THREE FREE THERAPIES

overtaxing the spleen *vis à vis* blood production. It is also a fact of life that the spleen typically becomes weak with age.

More importantly, chilled foods directly damage the spleen. Chilled, frozen foods and drinks neutralize the spleen's yang qi. The process of digestion is the process of turning all foods and drinks to 100° Fahrenheit soup within the stomach so that it may undergo distillation. If the spleen expends too much yang qi just warming the food up, then it will become damaged and weak. Therefore, all foods and liquids should be eaten and drunk at room temperature at the least and better at body temperature. The more signs and symptoms of spleen vacuity a person presents, such as fatigue, chronically loose stools, undigested food in the stools, cold hands and feet, dizziness on standing up, and aversion to cold, the more closely she should avoid uncooked, chilled foods and drinks.

In addition, sugars and sweets directly damage the spleen. This is because sweet is the flavor which inherently "gathers" in the spleen. It is also an inherently dampening flavor according to Chinese medicine. This means that the body engenders or secretes fluids which gather and collect, transforming into dampness, in response to foods with an excessively sweet flavor. In Chinese medicine, it is said that the spleen is averse to dampness. Dampness is yin and controls or checks yang qi. The spleen's function is based on the transformative and transporting functions of yang qi. Therefore, anything which is excessively dampening can damage the spleen. The sweeter a food is, the more dampening and, therefore, more damaging it is to the spleen.

Another group of foods which are dampening and, therefore, damaging to the spleen is what Chinese doctors call "sodden wheat foods." This means flour products such as bread and noodles. Wheat (as opposed to rice) is damp by nature. When wheat is steamed, yeasted, and/or refined, it becomes even more dampening. In addition, all oils and fats are damp by nature and, hence, may damage the spleen. The more oily or greasy a food is, the worse it is for the spleen. Because milk contains a lot of fat, dairy products are another spleen-damaging, dampness-engendering food. This includes milk, butter, and cheese.

If we put this all together, then ice cream is just about the worst thing a woman with a weak, damp spleen could eat. Ice cream is chilled, it is intensely sweet, and it is filled with fat. Therefore, it is a triple whammy when it comes to damaging the spleen. Likewise, pasta smothered in tomato sauce and cheese is a recipe for disaster. Pasta made from wheat flour is dampening, tomatoes are dampening, and cheese is dampening. In addition, what many people don't know is that a glass of fruit juice contains as much sugar as a candy bar, and, therefore, is also very damaging to the spleen and damp-engendering.

Below is a list of specific Western foods which are either uncooked, chilled, too sweet, or too dampening and thus damaging to the spleen. Persons with insomnia should minimize or avoid these proportional to how weak and damp their spleen is.

Ice cream	Juicy, sweet fruits, such as
Sugar	oranges, peaches, straw-
Candy, especially chocolate	berries, and tomatoes
Milk	Fatty meats
Butter	Fried foods
Cheese	Refined flour products
Margarine	Yeasted bread
Yogurt	Nuts
Raw salads	Alcohol (which is essentially
Fruit juices	sugar)

If the spleen is weak and wet, one should also not eat too much at any one time. A weak spleen can be overwhelmed by a large meal, especially if any of the food is hard-to-digest. This then results in food stagnation which only impedes the free flow of qi all the more and further damages the spleen.

A clear, bland diet

In Chinese medicine, the best diet for the spleen and, therefore, by extension for most humans, is what is called a "clear, bland diet." This is a diet high in complex carbohydrates such as unrefined grains, especially rice and beans. It is a diet which is high in *lightly cooked* vegetables. It is a diet which is low in fatty meats, oily, greasy, fried foods, and very sweet foods. However, it is not a completely vegetarian diet. Most people, in my experience should eat one to two ounces of various types of meat two to four times per week. This animal flesh may be the highly popular but over-touted chicken and fish, but should also include some lean beef, pork, and lamb. Some fresh or cooked fruits may be eaten, but fruit juices should be avoided. In addition, women should make an effort to include tofu and tempeh, two soy foods now commonly available in North American grocery food stores.

If the spleen is weak, then one should eat several smaller meals rather than one or two large meals. In addition, because rice is 1) neutral in temperature, 2) it fortifies the spleen and supplements the qi, and 3) it eliminates dampness, rice should be the main or staple grain in the diet.

A few problem foods

Coffee

There are a few "problem" foods which deserve special mention. The first of these is coffee. Many people crave coffee for two reasons. First, coffee moves stuck qi. Therefore, if a person suffers from liver depression qi stagnation, temporarily coffee will make them feel like their qi is flowing. Secondly, coffee transforms essence into qi and makes that qi temporarily available to the body. Therefore, people who suffer from spleen and/or kidney vacuity fatigue will get a temporary lift from coffee. They will feel like they have energy. However, once this energy is used up, they are left with a negative deficit. The coffee has transformed some of the essence stored in the kidneys into qi. This qi has been used, and now there is less stored essence. Since the blood and essence share a common source, coffee drinking may ultimately worsen insomnia associated with blood or kidney vacuities. Tea has a similar effect as coffee in that it transforms yin essence into yang qi and liberates that upward and outward through the body. However, the caffeine in black tea is usually only half as strong as in coffee.

Chocolate

Another problem food is chocolate. Chocolate is a combination of oil, sugar, and cocoa. We have seen that both oil and sugar are dampening and damaging to the spleen. Temporarily, the sugar will boost the spleen qi, but ultimately it will result in "sugar blues" or a hypoglycemic let down. Cocoa stirs the life gate fire. The life gate fire is another name for kidney yang or kidney fire, and kidney fire is the source of sexual energy and desire. It is said that chocolate is the food of love, and from the Chinese medical point of view, that is true. Since chocolate stimulates kidney fire at the same time as it temporarily boosts the spleen, it does give one rush of yang qi. In addition, this rush of yang qi does move depression and stagnation, at least short-term. So it makes sense that some people with liver depression, spleen vacuity, and kidney yang debility might crave chocolate.

Alcohol

Alcohol is both damp and hot according to Chinese medical theory. Hence, in English it is referred to as "fire water." It strongly moves the qi and blood. Therefore, persons with liver depression qi stagnation will feel temporarily better from drinking alcohol. However, the sugar in alcohol damages the spleen and engenders dampness which "gums up the works," while the heat (yang) in alcohol can waste the blood (yin) and aggravate or inflame depressive liver heat.

Hot, peppery foods

Spicy, peppery, "hot" foods also move the qi, thereby giving some temporary relief to liver depression qi stagnation. However, like alcohol, the heat in spicy hot foods wastes the blood and can inflame yang.

Sour foods

In Chinese medicine, the sour flavor is inherently astringing and constricting. Therefore, people with liver depression qi stagnation should be careful not to use vinegar and other intensely sour foods. Such sour flavored foods will only aggravate the qi stagnation by astringing and restricting the qi and blood all the more. This is also why sweet and sour foods, such as orange juice and tomatoes are particularly bad for people with liver depression and spleen vacuity. The sour flavor astringes and constricts the qi, while the sweet flavor damages the spleen and engenders dampness.

Diet sodas

In my experience, diet sodas seem to contain something that damages the Chinese idea of the kidneys. They may not damage the spleen the same way that sugared sodas do, but that does not mean they are healthy and safe. I say that diet sodas damage the kidneys since a number of my patients over the years have reported that, when they drink numerous diet sodas, they experience terminal dribbling, urinary incontinence, and low back and knee soreness and weakness. When they stop drinking diet sodas, these symptoms disappear. Taken as a group, in Chinese medicine, these are kidney vacuity symptoms. Since women in their late 30s and throughout their 40s tend to suffer from concomitant kidney vacuity (along with liver depression and spleen vacuity), I typically recommend such women to steer clear of diet sodas so as not to weaken their kidneys any further or faster. This also goes for men of any age who exhibit signs and symptoms of kidney vacuity.

Foods which help nourish the blood

Qi & Wei

According to Chinese dietary therapy, all foods contain varying proportions of qi and *wei*. Qi means the ability to catalyze or promote yang function, while *wei* (literally meaning flavor) refers to a food's ability to nourish or construct yin substance. Since blood is relatively yin compared to qi being yang, a certain amount of food high in *wei* is necessary for a person to engender and transform blood. Foods which are high in *wei* as compared to qi are those which tend to be heavy, dense, greasy or oily, meaty or bloody. All animal products contain more *wei* than vegetable products. At the same time, black beans or, even better, black soybeans contain more *wei* than celery or lettuce.

When people suffer from insomnia due to blood vacuity failing to nourish the heart and quiet the spirit or yin vacuity failing to control yang, they usually need to eat slightly more foods high in *wei*. This includes animal proteins and products, such as meat and eggs. It is said that flesh foods are very "compassionate" to the human body. This word recognizes the fact that the animal's life has had to be sacrificed to produce this type of food. It also recognizes that, because such food is so close to the human body itself, it is especially nutritious. Therefore, when people suffer from vacuity insomnia, eating some animal products usually is helpful and sometimes is down right necessary.

Animal foods vs. vegetarianism

Based on my many years of clinical experience, I have seen many Westerners adhering to a strict vegetarian diet develop, after several years, blood or yin vacuity patterns. This is especially the case in women who lose blood every month and must build babies out of the blood and yin essence. When women who are strict vegetarians come to me with various complaints, if they present the signs and symptoms of blood vacuity, such as a fat, pale tongue, pale face, pale nails, pale lips, heart palpitations, insomnia, and fatigue with a fine, forceless pulse, I typically recommend that they include a little animal food in their diet. In such cases, they commonly report to me how much better they feel immediately—how much more energy they have.

The downside of eating meat—besides the ethical issues—are that foods which are high in *wei* also tend to be harder to digest and tend to engender phlegm and dampness. Therefore, such foods should only be eaten in very small amounts at any one time. In addition, the weaker the person's spleen or the more phlegm and dampness they already have, the less such foods they should eat.

Remember above we said that the process of digestion first consisted of turning the food and drink ingested into 100° soup in the stomach. Therefore, soups and broths made out of animal flesh are the easiest and most digestible way of adding some animal-quality *wei* to a person's diet. When eating flesh itself, this should probably be limited to only one to two ounces per serving and only three or four such servings per week. According to Chinese dietary theory, the best foods for engendering and transforming blood and yin essence are organ meats and red or dark meats. This includes beef, buffalo, venison, and lamb and dark meat from chicken, turkey, goose, and duck. White meat fish and white meat fowl are less effective for building blood. However, white meat pork is also OK as is ham.

One good recipe for adding more digestible *wei* to the diet of a person who is blood vacuous is to take a marrow bone and boil this with some cut vegetables, especially root vegetables, and black beans or black soybeans. Such a marrow bone, black bean, and vegetable soup is easy to digest and yet rich in *wei*.

The proverbial glass of hot milk

The fact that milk is rich in *wei* is exactly why it is a soporific or sleep-inducer according to Chinese medicine. Being high in *wei* or yin, milk helps control counterflowing, hyperactive yang. Therefore, drinking some warm milk before bed-time is actually a good way to help insomnia *as long as the person does not suffer from either dampness or phlegm.* For persons with phlegm heat pattern insomnia, drinking a warm glass of milk before bed will typically make their insomnia worse! This is the beauty of Chinese medicine. It allows one to determine on an individual basis whether any food, medicine, or activity will be good for their particular pattern of imbalance. The Chinese would say that blending a whole egg into boiling milk makes this time-tested remedy even more effective for enriching yin.

The most important thing to remember about diet is that if: A) the spleen is healthy and strong, B) one eats primarily a clear, bland diet with a little bit of animal food, C) one gets sufficient exercise, but D) one does not overtax oneself, then one will manufacture good amounts of qi and blood. Whatever of this qi and blood is left unconsumed at the end of the day will be transformed into acquired essence that night. This is the safest way of engendering and transforming blood and yin via the diet. If one loads up on foods which are high in *wei*, in theory, these may supplement yin and nourish blood. However, if, in fact, they gum up the qi mechanism, the net result will be less qi and blood, not more, and one will have complicated their case even more by creating phlegm and dampness to boot.

In the following chapter, the reader will find some specific recipes combining Chinese herbs and foods for nourishing the blood and enriching yin, quieting the spirit and promoting sleep.

Some last words on diet

In conclusion, Western patients are always asking me what they should eat in order to cure their disease. However, when it comes to diet, sad to say, the issue is not so much what to eat as what not to eat. Diet most definitely plays a major role in the cause and perpetuation of many people's insomnia, but, except in the case of vegetarians suffering from blood or yin vacuities, the issue is mainly what to avoid or minimize, not what to eat. Most of us know that coffee, chocolate, sugars and sweets, oils and fats, and alcohol are not good for us. Most of us know that we should be eating more complex carbohydrates and freshly cooked vegetables and less fatty meats. However, it's one thing to know these things and another to follow what we know.

To be perfectly honest, a clear bland diet *à la* Chinese medicine is not the most exciting diet in the world. It is the traditional diet of most lower and lower middle class peoples around the world living in temperate climates. It is the traditional diet of most of my readers' great grandparents. The point I am making here is that our modern Western diet which is high in oils and fats, high in sugars and sweets, high in animal proteins, and proportionally high in uncooked, chilled foods and drinks is a relatively recent aberration, and you can't fool Mother Nature.

When one switches to the clear, bland diet of Chinese medicine, at first one may suffer from cravings for more "flavorful" food. These cravings are, in many cases, actually associated with food "allergies." In other words, we may crave what is actually not good for us similar to a drunk's craving alcohol. After a few days, these cravings tend to disappear and we may be amazed that we don't miss some of our convenience or "comfort" foods as much as we thought we would. If one has been addicted to a food like sugar for many years, it does not take much to "fall off the wagon" and be addicted again. Therefore, perseverance is the key to long-term success. As the Chinese say, a million is made up of nothing but lots of ones, and a bucket is quickly filled by steady drips and drops.

Exercise

Exercise is the second of what I call the three free therapies. According to Chinese medicine, regular and adequate exercise has two basic benefits. First, exercise promotes the movement of the qi and quickening of the blood. Since almost all insomnia involves at least some component of liver depression qi stagnation, it is obvious that exercise is an important therapy for coursing the liver and rectifying the qi. Secondly, exercise benefits the spleen. The spleen's movement and transportation of the digestate is dependent upon the qi mechanism. The qi mechanism describes the function of the qi in upbearing the pure and downbearing the turbid parts of digestion. For the qi mechanism to function properly, the qi must be flowing normally and freely. Since exercise moves and rectifies the qi, it also helps regulate and rectify the qi mechanism. This then results in the spleen's movement and transportation of foods and liquids and its subsequent engendering and transforming of the qi and blood. Because spleen and qi and blood vacuity typically complicate most people's insomnia and because a healthy spleen checks and controls a depressed liver, exercise treats one of the other commonly encountered disease mechanisms in the majority of Westerner's suffering from insomnia. Therefore, it is easy to see that regular, adequate exercise is a vitally important component of any person's regime for either preventing or treating insomnia.

What kind of exercise is best for insomnia?

Aerobics

In my experience, I find aerobic exercise to be the most beneficial for most people with insomnia. By aerobic exercise, I mean *any physical activity which raises one's heart beat 80% above their normal resting rate and keeps it there for at least 20 minutes.* To calculate your normal resting heart rate, place your fingers over the pulsing artery on the front side of your neck. Count the beats for 15 seconds and then multiply by four. This gives you your beats per minute or BPM. Now multiply your BPM by 0.8. Take the resulting number and add it to your resting BPM. This gives you your aerobic threshold of BPM. Next engage in any physical activity you like. After you have been exercising for five minutes, take your pulse for 15 seconds once again at the artery on the front side of your throat. Again multiply the resulting count by four and this tells you your current BPM. If this number is less than your aerobic threshold BPM, then you know you need to exercise harder or faster. Once you get your heart rate up to your aerobic threshold, then you need to keep exercising at the same level of intensity for at least 20 minutes. In order to insure that one is keeping their heart beat high enough for long enough, one should recount their pulse every five minutes or so.

Depending on one's age and physical condition, different people will have to exercise harder to reach their aerobic threshold than others. For some, simply walking briskly will raise their heart beat 80% above their resting rate. For others, they will need to do calisthenics, running, swimming, racket ball, or some other, more strenuous exercise. It really does not matter what the exercise is as long as it raises your heart beat 80% above your resting rate and keeps it there for 20 minutes. However, there are two other criteria that should be met. One, the exercise should be something that is not too boring. If it is too boring, then you may have a hard time keeping up your schedule. Since most people do find aerobic exercises such as running, stationary bicycles, and stair-steppers boring, it is good to listen to music or watch TV in order to distract your mind from the tedium. Secondly, the type of exercise should not cause any damage to any parts of the body. For instance, running on pavement may cause knee problems for some people. Therefore, you should pick a type of exercise you enjoy but also one which will not cause any problems.

When doing aerobic exercise, it is best to exercise either every day or every other day. If one does not do their aerobics at least once every 72 hours, then its cumulative effects will not be as great. Therefore, I recommend my patients with insomnia to do some sort of aerobic exercises every day or every other day, three to four times per week *at least*. The good news is that there is no real need to exercise more than 30 minutes at any one time. Forty-five minutes per session is not going to be all that much better than 25 minutes per session. And 25 minutes four times per week is very much better than one hour once a week.

Weight lifting

Recent research has also demonstrated that weight lifting can help relieve depression in women of all ages.[16] Insomnia is one of the important symptoms of depression, and certainly in clinic I see more women with insomnia than men. Therefore, I have begun recommending lifting weights on the days when one is not doing aerobics. In that case, one can do aerobics three to four days a

---

[16] "Depression and Weight Training", *Harvard Women's Health Watch*, Vol. IV, #6, February 1997, reporting on research published in the *Journal of Gerontology*, January 1997

week and lift weights the other three days. In general, one should not lift weights every day unless one varies the muscle groups they are working each day. In the study on weight lifting and depression cited above, the women lifted weights which were 45-87% as heavy as the maximum they could lift at one time. Those women who lifted weights closer to the top end of this range saw the greatest benefits. These women lifted weights three days per week for 10 weeks, gradually increasing the amount of weight they lifted at each session.

Because weight lifting requires some initial training and education in order to do safely and properly, I recommend taking a few classes either at a local YMCA or recreation center or from a private trainer. When aerobics are alternated with weight lifting, one has a really comprehensive training regime designed to benefit both one's cardiovascular system and one's muscles, tendons, ligaments, and bones. In addition, regular weight bearing exercise is also important for preventing osteoporosis.

Too much exercise

While the vast majority of people with insomnia will benefit from more exercise, there are a few who actually need less physical activity. As we have seen, all stirring or activity entails a consumption of yin by yang. If a person is either constitutionally yin vacuous or, due to some circumstance, like aging, enduring disease, extreme blood loss, excessive births, or lactation, has become yin vacuous, then too much exercise or physical activity can worsen that yin vacuity. This is mostly seen in women with thin bodily constitutions who over-exercise, such as professional athletes, or in women who suffer from anorexia and bulimia.

Body fat in Chinese medicine is nothing other than yin. Therefore, people who are very thinly built tend to have less yin to begin with. If, through exercise, one reduces their body fat even more, it may become so insufficient that yin can no longer control yang.

103

In women, such an insufficiency of yin blood due to over-consumption in turn due to too much exercise usually manifests itself first as cessation of menstruation or amenorrhea. However, it is also possible for drug use, especially types of "speed", or anorexia and bulimia to also result in an over consumption of yin leading to amenorrhea on the one hand and increased mental agitation and insomnia on the other. Here I am using the term bulimia as binging and purging, *i.e.*, eating but vomiting back up whatever has been ingested. Although the woman may be eating, often she still is not getting sufficient yin nourishment. It is also not uncommon to find an attraction to speed, a tendency to overexercise, and a tendency to anorexia all in the same woman.

In such women, it may be necessary to actually curtail the amount of exercise they are getting. One knows if the amount of exercise they are getting is a good amount if they feel refreshed and invigorated a couple of hours after the exercise is over. If, on the other hand, one feels even more fatigued or feels even more nervous and jittery, or if exercise during the day leads to night sweats and insomnia, then one should consider actually doing less exercise.

Deep relaxation

As we have seen above, insomnia is commonly associated with liver depression qi stagnation. If liver depression endures or is severe, it typically transforms into heat or fire. Heat or fire being yang, consume and exhaust yin and blood. Thus yang qi moves frenetically upward, disturbing the heart spirit. Therefore, liver depression is often at the root of insomnia. In Chinese medicine, liver depression comes from not fulfilling all one's desires. But as we have also seen above, no adult can fulfill all their desires. This is why a certain amount of liver depression is endemic among adults. When our desires are frustrated, our qi becomes depressed. This then creates emotional depression and easy anger or irritability. In Chinese medicine, anger is nothing other than the venting of pent up qi in the liver. When qi becomes depressed in the liver, it accumulates like hot air in a balloon. Eventually, that hot, depressed, angry qi has to go somewhere. So when there is a little more frustration or stress, then this angry qi in the liver vents itself as irritability, anger, shouting, or nasty words, and it moves upward in the body to disturb the spirit in the heart. In Chinese medicine, it is a basic statement of fact that, "Anger results in the qi ascending."

Essentially, this type of anger and irritability are due to a maladaptive coping response that is typically learned at a young age. When we feel frustrated or stressed, stymied by or angry about something, most of us tense our muscles and especially the muscles in our upper back and shoulders, neck, and jaws. At the same time, many of us will hold our breath. In Chinese medicine, the sinews are governed by the liver. This tensing of the muscles, i.e., the sinews, constricts the flow of qi in the channels and network vessels. Since it is the liver which is responsible for the coursing and discharging of this qi, such tensing of the sinews leads to liver depression qi stagnation. Because the lungs govern the downward spreading and movement of the qi, holding our breath due to stress or frustration only worsens this tendency of the qi not to move and, therefore, to become depressed in the Chinese medical idea of the liver.

Therefore, deep relaxation is the third of the three free therapies. For deep relaxation to be therapeutic medically, it needs to be more than just mental equilibrium. It needs to be somatic or bodily relaxation as well as mental repose. Most of us no longer recognize that every thought we think and feeling we feel is actually a felt physical sensation somewhere in our body. The words we use to describe emotions are all abstract nouns, such as anger, depression, sadness, and melancholy. However, in Chinese medicine, *every emotion is associated with a change in the direction or flow of qi*. As we have said above, anger makes the qi move upward. Fear, on the other hand, makes the qi move downward. Therefore, anger "makes our gorge rise" or "blow our top", while fear may cause a "sinking feeling" or make us "pee in our pants." These colloquial expressions are all based on the age-old wisdom that all thoughts and emotions are not just mental but also bodily events. This is why it is not just enough to clear one's mind. Clearing one's mind is good, but for really marked therapeutic results, it is even better if one clears one's mind at the same time as relaxing every muscle in the body.

Guided deep relaxation tapes

The single most efficient and effective way I have found for myself and my patients to practice such mental and physical deep relaxation is to do a daily, guided, progressive, deep relaxation audiotape. What I mean by guided is that a narrator on the tape leads one through the process of deep relaxation. Such tapes are progressive since they lead one through the body in a progressive manner, first relaxing one body part and then moving on to another. For instance, the narrator may say something to the effect that, as you exhale, you should feel your forehead get heavy and relaxed, softening and expanding, becoming warm and heavy. As you exhale again, now feel your cheeks get heavy and relaxed, softening and expanding, becoming warm and heavy. Breathe in and breathe out, letting your breath go without hindrance or hesitation. Breathing out, now feel your jaw muscles become heavy and relaxed, expanding and softening, becoming warm and heavy, etc., etc. throughout the entire body until one comes to the bottoms of one's feet.

There are innumerable such tapes on the market. These are usually sold in health food stores, New Age music and supply stores, or in bookstores with a good selection of New Age books. Over the years of suggesting this method of deep relaxation to my patients, I have found that each patient will have her own preferences in terms of the type of voice, male or female, the choice of words and imagery, whether there is background music or not, and the actual pace of the progression through the body, some narrators speaking a slightly different rate and rhythm. Therefore, I suggest listening to and even purchasing more than one such tape. One should find a tape which they like and can listen to without internal criticism or comment, going along like a cloud in the sky as the narrator's voice blows away all your mental and bodily stress and tension. If one has more than one tape, one can also switch every now and again from tape to tape so as not to become bored with the process or desensitized to the instructions.

Key things to look for in a good relaxation tape

In order to get the full therapeutic effect of such deep relaxation tapes, there are several key things to check for. First, be sure that the tape is a guided tape and not a subliminal relaxation tape. Subliminal tapes usually have music and any instructions to relax are given so quietly that they are not consciously heard. Although such tapes can help you feel relaxed when you do them, ultimately they do not teach you how to relax as a skill which can be consciously practiced and refined. Secondly, make sure the tape starts from the top of the body and works downward. Remember, anger makes the qi go upward in the body, and people with irritability and easy anger due to liver depression qi stagnation already have too much qi rising upward in their bodies. Such depressed qi typically needs not only to be moved but also downborne. Third, make sure the tape instructs you to relax your physical body. If you do not relax all your muscles or sinews, the qi cannot flow freely and the liver cannot be coursed. Depression is not resolved, and there will not be the same medically therapeutic effect. And lastly, be sure the tape instructs you to let your breath go with each exhalation. One of the symptoms of liver depression is a stuffy feeling in the chest which we then unconsciously try to relieve by sighing. Letting each exhalation go completely helps the lungs push the qi downward. This allows the lungs to control the liver at the same time as it downbears upwardly counterflowing angry liver qi.

The importance of daily practice

When I was an intern in Shanghai in the People's Republic of China, I was once taken on a field trip to a hospital clinic where they were using deep relaxation as a therapy with patients with high blood pressure, heart disease, stroke, migraines, and insomnia. The doctors at this clinic showed us various graphs plotting their research data on how such daily, progressive deep relaxation can regulate the blood pressure and body temperature and improve the appetite, digestion, elimination, sleep, energy, and mood. One of the things they said has stuck with me for 15 years: "Small results in 100 days, big results in 1,000." This means that if one does such daily, progressive deep relaxation *every single day for 100 days*, one will definitely experience certain results. What are these "small" results? These small results are improvements in all the parameters listed above: blood pressure, body temperature, appetite, digestion, elimination, sleep, energy, and mood. If these are "small" results, then what are the "big" results experienced in 1,000 days of practice? The "big" results are a change in how one reacts to stress—in other words, a change in one's very personality or character.

What these doctors in Shanghai stressed and what I have also experienced both personally and with my patients is that it is vitally important to do such daily, guided, progressive deep relaxation every single day, day in and day out for a solid three months at least and for a continuous three years at best. If one does such progressive, somatic deep relaxation every day, *one will see every parameter or measurement of health and well-being improve*. If one does this kind of deep relaxation only sporadically, missing a day here and there, it will feel good when you do it, but it will not have the marked, cumulative therapeutic effects it can.

108

Therefore, perseverance is the real key to getting the benefits of deep relaxation.

The real test

Doing such a daily deep relaxation regime is like hitting tennis balls against a wall or hitting a bucket of balls at a driving range. It is only practice; it is not the real game itself. Doing a daily deep relaxation regime is not only in order to relieve one's immediate stress and strain. It is to learn a new skill, a new way to react to stress. The ultimate goal is to learn how to breathe out and immediately relax all one's muscles in the body in reaction to stress, rather than the common but unhealthy maladaption to stress of holding one's breath and tensing one's muscles. By doing such deep relaxation day after day, one learns how to relax any and every muscle in the body quickly and efficiently. Then, as soon as one recognizes they are feeling frustrated, stressed out, or uptight, they can immediately remedy those feelings at the same time as coursing their liver and rectifying their qi. This is the real test, the game of life. "Small results in 100 days, big results in 1,000."

Finding the time

If you're like me and most of my patients, you are probably asking yourself right now, "All this is well and good, but when am I supposed to find the time to eat well-balanced cooked meals, exercise at least every other day, and do a deep relaxation every day? I'm already stretched to the breaking point." I know. That's the problem.

As a clinician, I often wish I could wave a magic wand over my patients' heads and make them all healthy and well. I cannot. After close to two decades of working with thousands of patients, I know of no easy way to health. There is good living and there is easy living. Or perhaps I am stating this all wrong. What most people take as the easy way these days is to continue pushing their limits continually to the max. The so-called path of least resistance is actually the path of lots and lots of resistance. Unless you take time for yourself and find the time to eat well, exercise, and relax, no treatment is going to eliminate your insomnia completely. There is simply no pill you can pop or food you can eat that will get rid of the root causes of insomnia: poor diet, too little exercise, and too much stress. Even Chinese herbal medicine and acupuncture can only get their full effect if the diet and lifestyle is first adjusted. Sun Si-maio, the most famous Chinese doctor of the Tang dynasty (618-907 CE), who himself refused government office and lived to be 101, said: "First adjust the diet and lifestyle and only secondarily give herbs and acupuncture." Likewise, it is said today in China, "Three parts treatment, seven parts nursing." This means that any cure is only 30% due to medical treatment and 70% is due to nursing, meaning proper diet and lifestyle.

In my experience, this is absolutely true. Seventy percent of all disease will improve after three months of proper diet, exercise, relaxation, and lifestyle modification. Seventy percent! Each of us has certain nondiscretionary rituals we perform each day. For instance, you may always and without exception find the time to brush your teeth. Perhaps it is always finding the time to shower. For others, it may be always finding the time each day to eat lunch. And for 99.999% of us, we find time, no, we make the time to get dressed each day. The same applies to good eating, exercise, and deep relaxation. Where there's a will there's a way. If your insomnia is bad enough, you can find the time to eat well, get proper exercise, and do a daily deep relaxation tape.

When it comes to daily deep relaxation and insomnia, the good news is that the right time is just before bed. Therefore, you do not have to find some other time to do this in the middle of your busy day. When you lie down at night, turn on your guided, progressive deep relaxation tape. If you are like most people,

110

either you will fall asleep even before the tape is finished or soon thereafter.

The solution to insomnia is in your hands

In Boulder, CO where I live, we have a walking mall in the center of town. On summer evenings, my wife and I often walk down this mall. Having treated so many patients over the years, it is not unusual for me to meet former patients on these strolls. Frequently when we say hello, these patients begin by telling me they are sorry they haven't been in to see me in such a long time. They usually say this apologetically as if they have done something wrong. I then usually ask if they've been alright. Often they tell me: "When my such-and-such flares up, I remember what you told me about my diet, exercise, and lifestyle. I then go back to doing my exercise or deep relaxation or I change my diet, and then my symptoms go away. That's why I haven't been in. I'm sorry."

However, such patients have no need to be sorry. This kind of story is music to my ears. When I hear that these patients are now able to control their own conditions by following the dietary and lifestyle advice I gave them, I know that, as a Chinese doctor, I have done my job correctly. In Chinese medicine, the inferior doctor treats disease after it has appeared. The superior doctor prevents disease before it has arisen. If I can teach my patients how to cure their symptoms themselves by making changes in their diet and lifestyle, then I'm approaching the goal of the high class Chinese doctor—the prevention of disease through patient education.

The professional practice of medicine is a strange business. We doctors are always or at least should be engaged in putting ourselves out of business. Therefore, patients have no need to

111

apologize to me when they tell me they now have in their own hands control over their health and disease.

To get these benefits, one must make the necessary changes in eating and behavior. In addition, insomnia is not a condition that is cured once and forever like measles or mumps. When I say Chinese medicine can cure insomnia, I do not mean that you will never experience unwanted wakefulness again. What I mean is that Chinese medicine can eliminate or greatly reduce your symptoms *as long as you keep your diet and lifestyle together*. People being people, we all "fall off the wagon" from time to time and we all "choose our own poisons." I do not expect perfection from either my patients or myself. Therefore, I am not looking for a lifetime cure. Rather, I try to give my patients an understanding of what causes their disease and what they can do to minimize or eliminate its causes and mechanisms. It is then up to the patient to decide what is bearable and what is unbearable or what is an acceptable level of health. The Chinese doctor will have done their job when *you know how to correct your health to the level you find acceptable given the price you have to pay.*

Simple Home Remedies for Insomnia

Although faulty diet, lack of adequate exercise, and too much stress are the ultimate causes of most insomnia according to Chinese medicine and, therefore, diet, exercise, and deep relaxation are the most important parts of every person's treatment and prevention of insomnia, there are a number of simple Chinese home remedies to help relieve the symptoms of insomnia, easy waking, and dream-disturbed sleep.

Regulating sleep & wake cycles

It is very common for someone who has had trouble either falling asleep or staying asleep to lay in bed in the morning in an effort to make up the sleep they lost at night. Although this seems like a common sense thing to do, it is actually not the right thing. When one sleeps later in the day to make up the sleep one lost the night before, this only further sets one's sleep-wake cycle back. Instead of feeling sleepy at one's normal bedtime, one will naturally stay awake later into the evening.

Therefore, I generally advise my insomniac patients not to lay in bed past their normal rising time in the morning. Yes, one probably will feel tired sooner in the day because of the lost sleep. However, that is exactly what the doctor ordered—well, wanted. It is also best, if possible, not to nap during the day if you are having trouble sleeping at night. This will likewise tend to reset one's sleep-wake cycle in a negative way. If one is able to go to sleep at the right time at night without difficulty, then a little nap is no problem. But if there is insomnia, it is best not to nap and not to lie about in bed in the mornings.

Chinese aroma therapy

In Chinese medicine, the qi is seen as a type of wind or vapor. The Chinese character for qi shows wind blowing over a rice field. In addition, smells are often referred to as a thing's qi. Therefore, there is a close relationship between smells carried through the air and the flow of qi in a person's body. Although aroma therapy has not been a major part of professionally practiced Chinese medicine for almost a thousand years, there is a simple aroma therapy treatment which one can do at home which can help alleviate premenstrual irritability, depression, nervousness, anxiety, and insomnia.

In Chinese, *Chen Xiang* means "sinking fragrance." It is the name of Lignum Aquilariae Agallochae or Eaglewood. This is a frequent ingredient in Asian incense formulas. In Chinese medicine, Aquilaria is classified as a qi-rectifying medicinal. When used as a boiled decoction or "tea", Aquilaria moves the qi and stops pain, downbears upward counterflow and regulates the middle (*i.e.*, the spleen and stomach), and promotes the kidneys' grasping of the qi sent down by the lungs. I believe that the word sinking in this herb's name refers to this medicinal's downbearing of upwardly counterflowing qi. Such upwardly counterflowing eventually must accumulate in the heart, disturbing and causing restlessness of the heart spirit. When this medicinal wood is burnt and its smoke is inhaled as a medicinal incense, its downbearing and spirit-calming function is emphasized.

One can buy Aquilaria or *Chen Xiang* from Chinese herb stores in Chinatowns, Japantowns, or Koreatowns in major urban areas. One can also buy it from Chinese medical practitioners who have their own pharmacies. It is best to use the powdered variety. However, powder may be made by putting a small piece of this aromatic wood in a coffee grinder. It is also OK to use small bits of the wood if powder is not available. Next one needs to buy a roll of incense charcoals. Place one charcoal in nonflammable dish and light it with a match. Then sprinkle a few pinches of Aquilaria powder on the lit charcoal. As the smoke rises, breathe in deeply. This can be done on a regular basis one or more times per day during the premenstruum or on an as-needed basis by those suffering from restlessness, nervousness, anxiety, irritability, and depression. For those who experience insomnia, one can do this "treatment" when laying in bed at night.

This Chinese aroma therapy with Lignum Aquilariae Agallochae is very cheap and effective. I know of no side effects or contra-indications.

Magnet therapy

The Chinese have used magnet therapy since at least the Tang dynasty (618-907 CE). Placing magnets on the body is a safe and painless way of stimulating acupuncture points without inserting needles through the skin. Since magnets can be taped onto points and "worn" for days at a time, Chinese magnet therapy is able to provide easy, low cost, continuous treatment. It is also possible to tape on magnets at night and to wear them to bed. Special adhesive magnets for stimulating acupuncture points, such as Accu-Band Magnets, Corimag, or Epaule Patch TDK Magnets, may be purchased from:

Oriental Medical Supply Co.
1950 Washington St. Braintree, MA 02184
Tel: (617) 331-3370 or 800-323-1839 Fax: (617) 335-5779

These magnets range in strength from 400-9,000 gauss, the unit measuring magnetic strength. For the treatments below, one can try 400-800 gauss magnets.

It is said in Chinese medicine that the ability to open and close the eyes has to do with the yang qi in two specific channels. These channels are called the *yin qiao mai* and the *yang qiao mai*. This translates as the yin and yang springing vessels. These two vessels both begin on the feet and meet at the eyes. The *yang qiao mai* carries yang qi upward to the head and specifically to the eyes. When this vessel is full of yang qi, the eyes are open and the person is awake. When this yang qi moves from the *yang qiao mai* into the *yin qiao mai* and is thence led back down into the lower and interior parts of the body, then the eyes close and one can go to sleep. Therefore, the yin and yang in the body that govern sleep and wake can be regulated by balancing the yin and yang qi in these two special vessels.

In most types of insomnia, yang qi is too full and is counterflowing upward out of control. In order to promote sleep, yin must be nourished in order to "magnetize" or attract yang to move back downward and inward. In insomnia, the yang qi in the *yang qiao mai* is too full or replete, while the yin qi in the *yin qiao mai* is vacuous and insufficient. In order to reestablish the balance between yin and yang in these two vessels, one needs to drain the *yang qiao mai* and supplement the *yin qiao mai*. In acupuncture, this can be done by using gold needles to supplement the meeting point of the *yin qiao mai* and silver needles to drain the *yang qiao mai*. It is also possible to drain these points with copper and zinc needles respectively. However, this requires puncturing the skin and should only be done by a professional acupuncturist.

Happily, one can get the same effect by taping small magnets over these points. The meeting or command point of the *yin qiao mai* is called *Zhao Hai* (Ki 6). It is located one inch beneath the tip of the inner ankle bone in a small depression below that bone. The meeting point of the *yang qiao mai* is called *Shen Mai* (Bl 62). It is located one inch below the tip of the outer ankle bone, also in a small depression. In order to drain the yang qi from *Shen Mai*, tape a small body magnet south side down over this point just before bed at night. In order to supplement the yin qi at *Zhao Hai*, tape a small body magnet north side down over that point just before bed at night. Do this to both sets of points on both feet.

116

Leave these magnets in place overnight, and remove them each morning when you wake. This can be done night after night until one is able to sleep without their aid.

Hydrotherapy

Hydrotherapy means water therapy and is also a part of traditional Chinese medicine. There are several different water treatments for helping relieve insomnia. First, let's begin with a warm bath. If one takes a warm bath (90-95°F) for 15-20 minutes, this can free and smooth the flow of qi and blood. In addition, it can calm the spirit and hasten sleep. Taking a warm bath a half hour before going to bed can help insomnia. When taking a warm bath to aid sleep, it is even more effective to put a cloth soaked in cold water on the forehead.

However, when using a warm bath, one must be careful not to use water so hot or to stay in the bath so long that sweat breaks out on one's forehead. Because "fluids and blood share a common source", excessive sweating can cause problems for women with blood and yin vacuities. Therefore, unless one is given a specific hot bath prescription by their Chinese medical practitioner, I suggest persons suffering from insomnia not stay in warm baths until they sweat. Although they may feel pleasantly relaxed, they may later feel excessively fatigued or excessively hot and thirsty. The later is especially the case in women who are peri-menopausal. In these women, hot baths may increase hot flashes and night sweats.

If, due to depression transforming heat, yang qi is exuberant and counterflowing upward, it may cause insomnia, migraines and tension headaches, hot flashes, night sweats, painful, red eyes, or even nosebleeds. In this case, one can tread in cold water up to their ankles for 15-20 minutes at a time. A variation of this is to fill one bucket with hot water (115°F) and another bucket with cold (60°F). First, dunk both feet in the hot water for three minutes, and then dunk them in the cold water for 30 seconds.

117

Alternate this procedure four times each treatment. Afterwards, dry the feet, put on warm socks, and go to bed. Another possibility is to soak heavy sweat socks in cold water and then put them on right before bed. Wrap these in plastic or a thick towel and remain in bed covered warmly. And the last hydrotherapy method is to soak a towel in cold water and use as a compress on the abdomen. Likewise, cover this compress with a plastic sheet or thick towel. All these treatments seek to draw yang qi away from the head to the lower part of the body.

Chinese self-massage

Massage, including self-massage, is a highly developed part of traditional Chinese medicine. The self-massage regime below is specifically designed as a home remedy for insomnia. For more Chinese self-massage regimes, the reader should see Fan Ya-li's *Chinese Self-massage Therapy: The Easy Way to Health* also published by Blue Poppy Press.

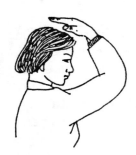

Begin by pressing and kneading the very center and top of the skull. This is acupoint *Bai Hui* (GV 20). It is the most yang point in the body and is the meeting place of all the yang channels and vessels. It is especially useful for calming the spirit, soothing the liver, and subduing hyperactive yang. Do this about 100 times.

Next, knead with the fingertips of both hands the acupoint located at the inner ends of the eyebrows. This area corresponds to the point *Zhan Zhu* (Bl 2). It is the place where the yang qi travelling up the *yang qiao mai* connects with the *yin qiao mai* which leads downward. Knead this area approximately 30 times.

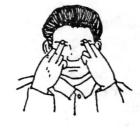

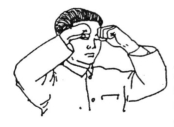

Third, with the index fingers and thumbs, wipe the upper edge of the eye bone and then the lower edge. Work from the inner corners of the eyes to the outer corners. This helps move the yang qi in the eyes downward and keeps it from congesting in the *yang qiao mai* in the eyes. Do this 20-30 times.

Fourth, rub the palms of the hands vigorously together until they feel warm. Then place these warm palms over both eyes. Cover the eyes thus for 30-60 seconds and then lightly rub the closed eyes approximately 10 times.

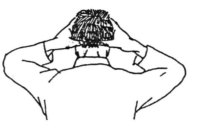

Fifth, press and knead the acupoint *Feng Chi* (GB 20) with the thumbs. This point is located in the depression between the mastoid process, the bone behind the ear, and the strap muscles on either side of the spine which connect at the base of the skull. The point is located approximately one inch within the hairline on most people. It is a point most people instinctively massage when they have a tension headache or stiff neck. Do this 30-50 times, massaging both points with both hands at the same time.

Sixth, rub circles around the center of the upper and then lower abdomen. The point in the middle of the upper abdomen is called *Zhong Wan* (CV 12). The point in the center of the lower abdomen is called *Guan Yuan* (CV 4). Rub these first clockwise and then counterclockwise approximately 100 times each point in each direction.

Seventh, press and kneading the acupoint *Nei Guan* (Per 6). This point is located on the inner side of the forearm in between the two tendons. It is located approximately 1.5 inches upward from

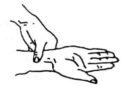

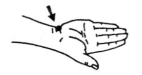

the wrist. First press and knead with the thumb of one hand, and then press and knead with the thumb of the other. Do this approximately 30-50 times on each side. This point helps soothe the liver, regulate the qi, and quiet the spirit.

Eighth, press and knead the point *Shen Men* (Ht 7). This is located on the inner side of the forearm at the crease of the wrist right below the base of the little or "pinky" finger. Massage the points on both wrists 30-50 times each. This point clears heat from the heart and quiets the spirit.

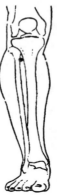

Now, press and knead the point *Zu San Li* (St 36). This point is located three inches below the lower, outside edge of the kneecap when the leg is bent. It is located in a depression between the muscles of the lower leg. Massage this point 30-50 times on each side. This point regulates the qi and leads upwardly counter-flowing yang qi downward.

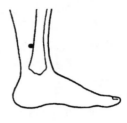

Follow this by pressing and kneading *San Yin Jiao* (Sp 6). This point is located three inches above the tip of the inner anklebone on the back side of the lower leg bone. It is the meeting place of the liver, spleen, and kidney channels. It is very effective for stimulating the production of yin blood in the body which can then "magnetize" yang qi back downward.

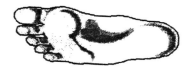

And lastly, rub the depression just behind and to the side of the ball of the foot. This point is called *Yong Quan* (Ki 1). If *Bai Hui* (GV 20) is the most yang point in the body, *Yong Quan* is the most yin.

Stimulating this point helps to lead counterflowing yang qi back downward to its lower source. Rub this point with the palm of the opposite hand until it feels hot. Repeat this on the other foot.

This self-massage regime should take between 20 minutes and one half hour. It should be done every evening just before bed. When doing each massage manipulation, you should try to calmly focus on the physical sensations under your hands and not let your mind wander to your day's worries and affairs.

Topical application of Chinese medicinals

Another safe and simple way of stimulating the healing properties of the acupuncture points is to apply Chinese medicinals to those points. The first such method for treating insomnia is to grind up 3-5g of Cinnabar (*Zhu Sha*) into powder. Make a paste with warm water and spread this on the point *Yong Quan* (Ki 1) described in the above Chinese self-massage protocol. Do this on both feet. Cinnabar is one of the famous spirit-quieting medicinals of Chinese medicine. Although this medicinal's internal use is debatable, its use externally is much safer. Apply this paste in the evening before bed and hold in place with an adhesive plaster. Remove this plaster and wash off in the morning on arising.

A second method is to grind 9g of Fructus Evodiae Rutecarpae (*Wu Zhu Yu*) into powder and mix into a paste with rice vinegar. Apply this paste over *Yong Quan* (Ki 1) on both sides. Do this before bed each night, and then remove and wash off this paste in the morning on arising.

121

And a third external application is to powder some Fructus Evodiae Rutecarpae (*Wu Zhu Yu*) and Cortex Cinnamomi Cassiae (*Rou Gui*). Mix this with some warm alcohol and make into a paste. Apply this paste before bed at night to *Yong Quan* (Ki 1) and remove in the morning.

Seven star hammering

A seven star hammer is a small hammer or mallet with seven small needles embedded in its head. Nowadays in China, it is often called a skin or dermal needle. It is one of the ways a person can stimulate various acupuncture points without actually inserting a needle into the body. Seven star hammers can be used either for people who are afraid of regular acupuncture, for children, or for those who wish to treat their condition at home. When the points to be stimulated are on the front of the body, this technique can be done by oneself. When they are located on the back of the body, this technique can be done by a family member or friend. This is a very easy technique which does not require any special training or expertise.

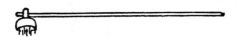

At least part of the seven star treatment for insomnia will require a helper. First, disinfect all the areas of the skin which are going to be tapped. Then begin by lightly tapping on the back of the neck. One should lightly tap all along the center of the spine on the neck as well as up and down the strap muscles to either side of the spinal column. Then one should lightly tap acupoints *Feng Chi* (GB 20). The location of these points behind the ear mastoid processes at the base of the skull has been described in the section on Chinese self-massage above. If one suffers from ascendant hyperactivity of liver yang, one can tap till the points bleed just a little bit. This helps drain heat or fire from the upper body. Otherwise tap until the skin is simply flushed red.

Next, tap all over the sacrum lightly until it turns a light red color. This is the triangular shaped bone at the base of the spine.

Follow this by tapping *Nei Guan* (Per 6), *Shen Men* (Ht 7), and *San Yin Jiao* (Sp 6) in that order. The locations of these three points have also been given under the section on Chinese self-massage above.

If there is headache due to ascendant hyperactivity of liver yang, tap over both temples. If the headache is severe, tap till just a little blood is let.

If there is any bleeding, wipe the area with a cotton swab moistened in alcohol or hydrogen peroxide. Then take a dry cotton ball and press the area. Between treatments, soak the seven star hammer in alcohol or hydrogen peroxide and do not share hammers between people in order to prevent any infection from one person to another. Seven star hammers are very cheap. So each person can easily afford to have their own. They can also be purchased from Oriental Medical Supply Co. whose address and phone numbers are given in the section on Chinese magnet therapy above.

Chinese medicinal wines

Chinese medicinal wines are part of Chinese dietary therapy. They make use of alcohol's special characteristics as well as a few Chinese herbs or medicinals. Although alcohol is hot and can inflame yang heat, especially liver heat, alcohol moves depressed qi and static blood. It also speeds and increases the medicinal effects of herbs into and in the body. Therefore, one can cautiously make and take a number of simple Chinese medicinal wines for the self-treatment of insomnia.

If there is liver blood-kidney yin vacuity, then the treatment principles are to supplement the kidneys and nourish the liver. This can be done by soaking 150g of Fructus Lycii Chinensis (*Gou*

Qi Zi) in one quart or fifth of brandy for 1-2 months. After the herbs have soaked, one can remove the dregs and then take 1-2 ounces each night before bed. Another possibility is to soak 150g of Radix Polygoni Multiflori in one quart or fifth of brandy for a couple of months. Later, remove the dregs, and take 1-2 ounces before or after dinner. Do not use this Chinese medicinal wine if there is diarrhea or chronically loose stools.

For heart blood-spleen qi vacuity insomnia, one can try either of two self-made Chinese medicinal wines. The first is made by placing 150g of white Ginseng (Radix Panacis Ginseng, *Ren Shen*) in one quart or fifth of brandy for 1-2 months. Then remove the dregs, and take 1-2 ounces before or after dinner. However, do not use this wine if you display the signs and symptoms of ascendant hyperactivity of liver yang. One can also use 150g of Arillus Euphoriae Longanae (*Long Yan Rou*) steeped in one quart or fifth of sake. In that case, drink 1-2 ounces before or after dinner each evening. Do not take this latter wine if you suffer from constipation.

For insomnia due to phlegm blocking or confounding the portals of the heart, take 120g of Rhizoma Acori Graminei (*Shi Chang Pu*) and soak this in one quart or fifth of vodka for 3-5 days. Then take 10-20ml of the resulting medicinal wine three times per day on an empty stomach.

These are only a few of the Chinese medicinal wines and elixirs that can be made and used at home for the treatment of insomnia. For more information on this subject, the reader may see my *Chinese Medical Wines & Elixirs* also published by Blue Poppy Press.

Chinese medicinal porridges

Like the Chinese medicinal wines discussed above, Chinese medicinal porridges are a specialized part of Chinese dietary therapy. Because porridges are already in the form of 100° soup, they are a particularly good way of eating otherwise nutritious but nevertheless hard to digest grains. When Chinese medicinals are cooked along with those grains, one has a high-powered but easily assimilable "health food" of the first order.

For yin vacuity insomnia, boil 60g of Bulbus Lilii (*Bai He*) along with 100g of white rice. Add a little brown sugar to taste and eat one time each day for 10 days. Another medicinal porridge for treating yin vacuity insomnia can be made by first boiling 50g of uncooked Radix Rehmanniae (*Sheng Di*) and 50g of Semen Zizyphi Spinosae (*Suan Zao Ren*) into a "tea" for 30-45 minutes. Then use this "tea" to boil 100g of white rice into a gruel. Eat this as often as one pleases on a daily basis.

For heart blood-spleen qi vacuity insomnia, cook 100g of white rice with 50g of Semen Coicis Lachryma-jobi (*Yi Yi Ren*) and 10 red dates (Fructus Zizyphi Jujubae, *Da Zao*). Eat this one time per day. Another recipe is to cook 50g of Sclerotium Poriae Cocos (*Fu Ling*) with 100g of white rice with enough water to make a thin porridge or gruel.

For numerous more Chinese medicinal porridge formulas for insomnia, see my *The Book of Jook, Chinese Medicinal Porridges: A Healthy Alternative to the Typical Western Breakfast* also published by Blue Poppy Press.

Chinese medicinal teas

Chinese medicinal teas may be seen as either Chinese herbal medicine or as Chinese dietary therapy. They consist of using only one or two Chinese herbal medicinals in order to make a tea which is then drunk as one's beverage throughout the day. Such Chinese medicinal teas are usually easier to make and better tasting than multi-ingredient, professionally prescribed decoctions. They can be used as an adjunct to professional prescribed Chinese herbs or as an adjunct to acupuncture or other Chinese therapies for insomnia.

For yin and blood vacuity insomnia, grind 15g of Semen Biotae Orientalis (*Bai Zi Ren*) into pieces. Boil with water and add honey to taste. Drink either before or after dinner. Or boil 15g of Fructus Mori Albi (*Sang Shen*) in water. Remove the dregs and drink one packet per day.

For phlegm obstruction with liver yang hyperactivity, *i.e.*, gallbladder timidity, grind Rhizoma Acori Graminei (*Shi Chang Pu*), 6g, Flos Jasmini (*Mo Li Hua*), 6g, and green tea, 10g, into coarse powder. Soak some of this powder in boiling water and drink as a tea any time of the day. The doses given are for a one day's supply. Another formula for gallbladder timidity consists of Dens Draconis (*Long Chi*), 10g, and Rhizoma Acori Graminei (*Shi Chang Pu*), 3g. First boil the Dens Draconis in water for 10 minutes. Then add the Rhizoma Acori Graminei and continue boiling for another 10-15 minutes. Remove the dregs and drink any time of the day, 1-2 packets per day.

For fire disturbing the heart spirit, boil 60g each of Medulla Junci Effusi (*Deng Xin Cao*) and Folium Lophatheri Gracilis (*Dan Zhu Ye*). Remove the dregs and drink the resulting tea warm at any time of the day, one packet per day.

For more information on Chinese medicinal teas, see Zong Xiao-fan and Gary Liscum's *Chinese Medicinal Teas: Simple, Proven, Folk Formulas for Common Diseases & Promoting Health* also published by Blue Poppy Press.

The medicinals in all the formulas in this chapter can be purchased by mail from:

China Herb Co.
165 W. Queen Lane
Philadelphia, PA 19144
Tel: 215-843-5864 Fax: 215-849-3338 Orders: 800-221-4372

When using any Chinese medicinal in any form, if there are any side effects, stop immediately and seek a consultation with a professional practitioner of Chinese medicine.

Flower therapy

People have been giving other people flowers for millennia to help them feel good. In Chinese medicine, there is actually a practice of flower therapy. Because the beauty of flowers bring most people joy and because joy is the antidote to the other four or six negative emotions of Chinese medicine,[17] flowers can help promote the free and easy flow of qi. It is said in Chinese medicine that, "Joy leads to relaxation (in the flow of qi)", and relaxation is exactly what the doctor ordered in the case of insomnia. As Wu Shi-ji wrote in the Qing dynasty, "Enjoying flowers can divert a person from their boredom and alleviate suffering caused by the seven affects (or emotions)."

However, there is more to Chinese flower therapy than the beauty of flowers bringing joy. Flower therapy also includes aroma-therapy. A number of Chinese medicinals come from plants which have flowers used in bouquets. For instance, Chrysanthemum flowers (*Ju Hua*, Flos Chrysanthemi Morifolii) are used to calm the liver and clear depressive heat rising to the upper body. The aroma of Chrysanthemum flowers thus also has a salutary, relaxing, and cooling effect on liver depression and depressive heat. Rose (*Mei Gui Hua*, Flos Rosae Rugosae) is used in Chinese medicine to move the qi and quicken the blood. Smelling the fragrance of Roses also does these same things. Other flowers used in Chinese medicine to calm the spirit and relieve stress and irritability are Lily, Narcissus, Lotus flowers, Orchids, and Jasmine. And further, taking a smell of a bouquet of flowers promotes deep breathing, and this, in turn, relieves pent up qi in

---

[17] In Chinese medicine, the emotions are sometimes counted as five and sometimes counted as seven. When counted as seven, fright and melancholy are added to anger, joy, thinking, sorrow, and fear.

the chest at the same time as it promotes the flow of qi downward via the lungs.

Creating a personalized regime

One does not need to do all these home treatments for every case of insomnia. Rather, one should select several of them as the severity of their disease, time, and personal inclination suggest. If one is already taking care of the Three Free Therapies, it is easy to add Chinese aroma therapy, Chinese magnet therapy, Chinese flower therapy, and a choice of Chinese medicinal teas, wines, and/or porridges. If one does not have access to body magnets, then one might switch this home therapy for Chinese hydrotherapy instead, or one might choose Chinese self-massage therapy. If one doesn't have the patience or discipline to do Chinese self-massage, but a partner is willing to do seven star hammering, then one might choose this therapy instead of either hydrotherapy or self-massage. In other words, it all depends on how severe the insomnia is and what materials one has at one's disposal.

Given the several different Chinese self-therapies in this chapter, no one should be unable to find the materials or the time to put at least one of these into practice. In some light cases of insomnia, that may be all it takes. While in more difficult, stubborn cases, one may have to do a couple or three of these to insure a good night's sleep without side effects or morning after grogginess.

Kicking the Sedative Habit

Some readers may be currently using Western sleep medications. These may be either over-the-counter nostrums or prescription sedatives and "tranquilizers." In general, it is not a good idea to discontinue such medications abruptly without checking with your Western physician. Your Western physician will be able to tell you whether or not you can stop taking a medication immediately or whether it needs to be tapered off at a certain schedule.

It is best if your Western MD and your Chinese medical practitioner can work hand in hand. Therefore, if you are currently taking any Western medication, whether prescription or over-the-counter, it is important to tell your Chinese medical practitioner what you are taking. In general, there is no problem with taking Western sedatives and tranquilizers with Chinese medicinals or at the same time as receiving acupuncture for insomnia. If anything, the Chinese medical treatment will make the Western medicines work better and with less side effects. What you should notice fairly quickly is that you need to take less and less of your Western medications to achieve the same or even better ability to go and stay asleep. Thus acupuncture and Chinese medicinals can actually help you get off Western sedatives and tranquilizers at the same time as addressing the root of your insomnia.

In particular, ear acupuncture has been used all over the U.S.A. to help people kick drug and alcohol addictions. Because press needles can be embedded in the ear between regularly scheduled office visits, this technique allows the calming therapy of acupuncture to exert a continuous effect. Therefore, using ear acupuncture, one can typically avoid any rebound jitters or nervousness when cutting down or stopping taking Western sedatives and tranquilizers.

However, readers who may be suffering from severe mental problems, such as schizophrenia or bi-polar disorder (a.k.a. manic depressive disorder), *should not stop taking their Western medication.* Acupuncture and Chinese medicine may help relieve any unwanted side effects from such Western medication, but typically are not sufficient by themselves for treating such sever mental-emotional problems. Likewise, anyone suffering from severe depression with any thoughts of suicide should immediately seek help from a qualified Western physician or psychotherapist.

12

Chinese Medical Research on Insomnia

Considerable research has been done in the People's Republic of China on the effects of acupuncture and Chinese herbal medicine on insomnia. Usually, this research is in the form of a clinical audit. That means that a group of patients with the same diseases, patterns, or major complaints are given the same treatment for a certain period of time. After this time, the patients are counted to see how many were cured, how many got a marked effect, how many got some effect, and how many got no effect. This kind of "outcome-based research" has, up until only very recently, not been considered credible in the West where, for the last 30 years or so, the double-blind, placebo-controlled comparison study has been considered the "gold standard." However, such double-blind, placebo-controlled comparison studies are impossible to design in Chinese medicine and do not, in any case, measure effectiveness in a real-life situation.

Clinical audits, on the other hand, do measure actual clinical satisfaction of real-life patients. Such clinical audits may not exclude the patient's trust and belief in the therapist or the therapy as an important component in the result. However, real-life is not as neat and discreet as a controlled laboratory experiment. If the majority of patients are satisfied with the results of a particular treatment and there are no adverse side effects to that treatment, then that is good enough for the Chinese doctor, and, in my experience, that is also good enough for the vast majority of my patients.

Below are abbreviated translations of several recent research articles published in Chinese medical journals on the treatment of insomnia. These research articles exemplify how Chinese medicine treats one of the most common yet distressing complaints. I think that most persons reading these statistics would think that Chinese medicine was worth a try. Even better results can be expected when treatments are even more finely tuned to the individual patient as is the case in private practice here in the West.

"The Treatment of 22 Cases of Insomnia in Young Adults Mainly by Acupuncturing *Si Shen Cong* (M-HN-1)" by Piao Ming-hua, *Hei Long Jiang Zhong Yi Yao (Heilongjiang Chinese Medicine & Medicinals)*, 1995, #6, p. 38-39

All 22 patients in this clinical audit were seen as outpatients. There were 12 females and 10 males. The youngest was 11 years old and the oldest was 28. The shortest course of disease was seven days and the longest was four years. Eighteen cases had already been administered Western sedatives. Either these had not produced a markedly good effect or they had caused side effects. The author mentions that insomnia in young adults is mostly due to overtaxation and thinking too much.

The treatment method mainly consisted of needling *Si Shen Cong* (M-HN-1). If there was heart-spleen detriment and decline, *Xin Shu* (Bl 15), *Pi Shu* (Bl 20), and *Jue Yin Shu* (Bl 14) were added. If heart and kidneys were not interacting, *Xin Shu* (Bl 15), *Shen Shu* (Bl 23), and *Tai Xi* (Ki 3) were added. If there was heart-gallbladder vacuity and timidity, *Xin Shu* (Bl 15), *Dan Shu* (Bl 19), and *Da Ling* (Per 7) were added. If there was spleen-stomach disharmony, *Wei Shu* (Bl 21) and *Zu San Li* (St 36) were added. And if there was ascendant hyperactivity of liver yang, *Gan Shu* (Bl 18), *Jian Shi* (Per 5), and *Tai Chong* (Liv 3) were added. The needles were left in place for 30 minutes and were stimulated once every 10 minutes. One treatment was given per day and 10 treatments equalled one course of therapy. After one course, the patient was allowed to rest for 3-5 days before starting a new course of therapy.

Supplementally, in order to strengthen the treatment effect and depending on the patient's pattern and signs and symptoms, small seeds or pellets were taped to one or more of the following ear acupuncture points: *Shen Men* (Spirit Gate), Subcortex, Heart, Liver, Spleen, or Kidneys. Up to six of these ear points were selected. The patient was instructed to press each of these pellets four times each day in order to stimulate these points. The points were pressed before sleep, after waking, in the morning, and in the afternoon. Both ears were treated at the same time.

Cure was defined as being able to go to sleep easily and staying asleep for seven hours or more. Marked effect meant that one could go to sleep relatively easily and could stay asleep for more than five hours. Some effect meant that the symptoms were decreased but the condition relapsed. No effect meant that the condition was the same as before treatment. Based on these criteria, after two whole courses of therapy, 14 cases or 63.64% were cured; five cases or 22.73% got a marked effect; and three cases or 22.73% got some effect. Therefore, the total effectiveness rate was 100%. Further, more than half these cases took an obvious turn for the better after a single treatment.

"Joining Needling at *Nei Guan* (Per 6) in the Treatment of 202 Cases of Insomnia" by Liu Bing-quan, *Xin Zhong Yi* (New Chinese Medicine), #5, 1996, p. 34

Of the 202 patients studied in this clinical audit, 82 were male and 120 were female. Their ages ranged from 18-65, with the majority being between 30-45 years old. In 54 cases, their course of disease has lasted six months to one year. In 128 cases, it had lasted one to three years. And in 20 cases, it had lasted for more than three years. Eighty-five percent of these patients continued to take or intermittently took sleeping medications. These 202 patients were divided into two groups of 101 patients each for comparison purposes.

In terms of their diagnostic criteria, these patients all suffered from inability to go to sleep, difficulty going to sleep, sometimes sleeping and sometimes being aroused, difficulty sleeping after being aroused, or sleep diminished by 40%. In some cases, they could only go to sleep after taking sleeping medication. Most of these patients also had varying degrees of dizziness, headache, heart palpitations, and impaired memory.

In one group, called the Needling *Nei Guan* Group, the treatment method consisted of acupuncturing *Nei Guan* (Per 6) to a depth of 0.8-1 inch deep along with the points *Shen Men* (Ht 7) and *Tai Chong* (Liv 3). In the second group, called the Joining Needling *Nei Guan* Group, *Nei Guan* was needled deeply through to *Wai Guan* (TB 5) but without breaking the skin on the opposite side of the forearm. After obtaining the needling sensation the needles were stimulated one time every 10 minutes with even supplementing/even draining technique. The needles were retained for 30 minutes per treatment with one treatment given per day. Thirty such treatments equalled one course of therapy.

Patients were considered cured if their sleep increased to 70-80% per night or more and they could stop taking sleeping medication. Marked effect meant that sleep increased to 60-70% and they could stop taking sleeping medication. Some effect meant that sleep increased to 50-60% per night and they could stop taking sleeping medication. No effect meant that sleep per night was only 40% or below and patients had to continue taking their sleeping medication.

Based on these criteria, in the Joining Needling Group, 35 cases were cured, 34 got a marked effect, 20 got some effect, and 12 got no effect. Thus the total improvement rate for this group was 88.1%. In the *Nei Guan* Group, 20 were cured, 16 got marked effect, 40 got some effect, and 25 got no effect. Therefore, the total improvement rate in this group was 75.2%. Thus both these treatments were considered statistically significantly effective.

"A Survey of the Treatment Efficacy of Treating Recalcitrant Insomnia with *Xue Fu Zhu Yu Tang* (Blood Mansion Dispel Stasis Decoction)" by Zhan Guo-tong, *Xin Zhong Yi (New Chinese Medicine)*, 1996, #8, p. 32-33

Of the 31 patients in this clinical audit, 26 were outpatients and five were inpatients. There were 11 males and 20 females. Three were between 15-30 years of age; eight were between 31-40; eight were between 41-50; nine were between 51-60, and three were 61 years old or older. Their course of disease had lasted six months to one year in five cases, from one to five years in 17 cases, from five to ten years in seven cases, and for more than 10 years in two cases.

All the patients in this study exhibited varying degrees of blood stasis, such as piercing pain in the head, dizziness, static macules on their tongues, and a choppy pulse. In addition, four other patterns were also discriminated: qi vacuity and blood stasis (11 cases), blood vacuity and blood stasis (8 cases), yin vacuity and blood stasis (6 cases), and phlegm heat and blood stasis (6 cases).

Based on everyone in this study suffering from blood stasis as at least part of the mechanisms of their insomnia, *Xue Fu Zhu Yu Tang* (Blood Mansion Dispel Stasis Decoction) was used as the guiding prescription. This was then modified for each of the four complicating patterns. The basic formula consisted of: Semen Pruni Persicae (*Tao Ren*), Flos Carthami Tinctorii (*Hong Hua*),

135

Radix Angelicae Sinensis (*Dang Gui*), Fructus Citri Aurantii (*Zhi Ke*), Radix Rubrus Paeoniae Lactiflorae (*Chi Shao*), Radix Platycodi Grandiflori (*Jie Geng*), 10g @, uncooked Radix Rehmanniae (*Sheng Di*), 15g, Radix Achyranthis Bidentatae (*Niu Xi*), 6g, Caulis Polygoni Multiflori (*Ye Jiao Teng*), 30g, Succinum (*Hu Po*), 1.5g, uncooked Radix Glycyrrhizae (*Gan Cao*), 3g.

If there was concomitant qi vacuity, Radix Codonopsitis Pilosulae (*Dang Shen*), 10g, and mix-fried Radix Astragali Membranacei (*Huang Qi*), 50g, were added. If there was concomitant blood vacuity, cooked Radix Rehmanniae (*Shu Di*), 25g, and Gelatinum Corii Asini (*E Jiao*), 10g, were added. If there was simultaneous yin vacuity, Fructus Lycii Chinensis (*Gou Qi Zi*), 15g, Fructus Corni Officinalis (*Shan Zhu Yu*), 12g, Rhizoma Acori Graminei (*Shi Chang Pu*), 6g, Radix Polygalae Tenuifoliae (*Yuan Zhi*), 5g, Radix Glehniae Littoralis (*Bei Sha Shen*), and Tuber Ophiopogonis Japonici (*Mai Dong*), 10g @, were added. If there was simultaneous phlegm heat, Pericarpium Citri Reticulatae (*Chen Pi*), 10g, Rhizoma Pinelliae Ternatae (*Ban Xia*) and processed Rhizoma Arisaematis (*Nan Xing*), 12g @, and Radix Scutellariae Baicalensis (*Huang Qin*) and Tuber Curcumae (*Yu Jin*), 10g @, were added. These were decocted in water and administered, one packet per day in two divided doses, morning and evening.

Cure meant that the patients were able to easily fall asleep each evening and sleep for eight hours or more. In addition, all their other symptoms disappeared. Marked effect meant that patients could sleep for at least six hours each evening and the major part of their accompanying symptoms disappeared. Some effect meant that the patient's sleep each night was longer than before. However, it still remained less than six hours. Or it meant that some of their symptoms disappeared. No effect meant that there was no change for the better in sleep and no improvement in symptoms.

Based on the above criteria, of the patients in the qi vacuity pattern group, six were cured, three registered marked improvement, and two got some effect. In the yin vacuity group, three were cured, two registered marked improvement, and one got some effect. Of the patients in the blood vacuity group, six were cured and two registered marked improvement. And of those in the phlegm heat group, one was cured, three got some effect, and two got no effect. Therefore, using this protocol, those patients in the blood vacuity/blood stasis group got the best results and those in the phlegm heat/blood stasis group got the worst. Twenty-four cases were followed up from one to three years, and only two cases had relapses. The cure rate was 51.6% and the total effectiveness rate was 93.5%.

"The Treatment of 12 Cases of Recalcitrant Insomnia by Tapping the Governing Vessel" by Zhuang Dan-hong, *Hei Long Jiang Zhong Yi Yao (Heilongjiang Chinese Medicine & Medicinals)*, 1996, #3, p. 47

Eight of the patients in this study were male and four were female. All were young, seemingly healthy adults. Ten cases suffered from overtaxation due to too much study and "brain work." Two cases were workers. The treatment method consisted of first disinfecting the skin over the vertebrae from the neck to the sacrum. Then a small hammer with several small needles embedded in its head was used to tap up and down over the governing vessel on the midline of the back. This tapping was continued until either the area tapped was flushed red or there was very, very slight bleeding. This was done one time each day. All the patients in this study were cured using this technique.

By way of example, the author gives a case history. The patient was a 34 -ear old male who worked as a teacher. He had suffered from recurrent insomnia for four years which was lately even more severe. He had difficulty falling asleep, dizziness, heart palpitations, lack of strength of his entire body, poor appetite, constipation, reddish colored urine, a red tongue with yellow fur, and a fine, rapid pulse. He had previously been administered a couple of different Chinese herbal decoctions which had not proven particularly effective. This had been combined with oral administration of Western sleep medication which had put him to sleep. When he decided to come to the hospital for acupuncture treatment he had stopped taking these sleep medications and he was only sleeping approximately three hours per night. After being treated with the above protocol two-three times, his sleep increased to four to five hours. He stopped taking the Chinese medicinals and his treatment was stabilized after three more treatments, at which time he was discharged from the hospital.

The author says that insomnia is mostly due to yin vacuity with yang hyperactivity. Tapping the governing vessel like this regulates yin and yang, rectifies the qi and blood, harmonizes the viscera and bowels, and frees the flow of the channels and network vessels. When the tapping causes a little bleeding, it further drains yang heat which is hyperactive and exuberant. This then has the effect of levelling or calming yin and secreting yang. As it is said, "When yin is levelled and yang secreted, the essence spirit [i.e., the mind] is treated [i.e., cured]."

More Case Histories

In order to help readers get a better feel for how Chinese medicine treats insomnia, I have given below some more case histories. These are the stories of real-life people who have been treated with acupuncture and/or Chinese medicine for insomnia and have gotten a good effect. Hopefully, you will be able to see yourself and your symptoms in these stories and be encouraged to give acupuncture and Chinese medicine a try.

Gary

Gary was a 34 year-old publisher whose chief complaint was insomnia. Three months before coming in, he had been assigned to oversee a very important job with a very tight deadline. Therefore, he had worked round the clock for one whole week. As a result of this intense mental and physical strain, he found it progressively harder and harder to fall asleep. Most nights he would toss and turn for three-four hours before finally sinking into the "sweet balm" of sleep. However, once asleep, he was disturbed by excessive dreams and was easily awakened. On really bad nights, Gary was only able to sleep for two-three hours. Then, the next day, he felt tired and dizzy and particularly weak in his low back region and knees.

When Gary was questioned, his Chinese doctor found out that he had been suffering from frequent night sweats along with the insomnia and that he was now plagued with premature ejaculation when he had sex with his girlfriend. He had tried some Western tranquilizers. If he took the prescribed dose, they didn't work, but if he took a double dose, he was groggy and couldn't think straight all the next day. Recently, he had rearranged his work schedule and tried to relax. But, so far, his insomnia had not improved. On examination, Gary's tongue had a red tip with thin fur, while his pulse felt thready.

Gary's Chinese pattern discrimination was loss of interaction between the heart and kidneys. Therefore, the treatment principles were to restore the interaction between the heart and kidneys by nourishing kidney yin, clearing heat fire, and leading yang back to its lower source. Gary was given the following Chinese medicinal prescription:

cooked Radix Rehmanniae (*Shu Di*), 12g
Radix Dioscoreae Oppositae (*Shan Yao*), 9g
Fructus Corni Officinalis (*Shan Zhu Yu*), 9g
Sclerotium Poriae Cocos (*Fu Ling*), 9g
Fructus Schisandrae Chinensis (*Wu Wei Zi*), 9g
Cortex Radicis Moutan (*Dan Pi*), 9g
Rhizoma Alismatis (*Ze Xie*), 9g
Cortex Cinnamomi Cassiae (*Rou Gui*), 6g
Rhizoma Coptidis Chinensis (*Huang Lian*), 3g

The above Chinese medicinals were decocted in water and administered in two divided doses per day after lunch and dinner. In addition, Gary was instructed on how to tape magnets over *Shen Mai* (Bl 62) and *Zhao Hai* (Ki 6) before bed each night. He was told to stay away from hot, spicy food, fried, fatty foods, alcohol, and all stimulants such as coffee, tea, or chocolate.

After taking the above Chinese medicinals, Gary returned to the clinic to report that he was now sleeping five or more hours each night and that he fell asleep easily within a half hour of going to bed. After two weeks' administration of the above formula, he was able to sleep normally throughout the night, getting a full seven hours sleep. On inspection, his tongue no longer had a red tip and his other symptoms had all markedly improved.

Priscilla

Priscilla was 52 years old. She had been suffering from insomnia for two years. This had begun shortly after her menstruation had ceased for good. Like Gary, Priscilla also had night sweats along with her insomnia. Although Priscilla had some trouble going to sleep, her real difficulty was staying asleep. She would typically sleep for four hours and then wake without being able to go back to sleep. Thus, she would toss and turn restlessly until daybreak when she would get up and go on about her day.

Besides matitudinal insomnia and night sweats, Priscilla had hot flashes during the day. She would not only feel flushed in the face, but the palms of her hands and soles of her feet would feel hot. However, at night her feet would be cold as ice. When she woke up in the early morning hours, it was typically to urinate. All her life she had been able to sleep through the night without having to go to the bathroom, but now she would urinate at least once and often two times each night. In addition, Priscilla complained of a chronically sore low back and no interest in sex whatsoever. This latter was also a change from before menopause, and a change her husband certainly wasn't happy about. On inspection, Priscilla's tongue also had a red tip, but its body was paler than normal and its fur was scanty and dry. Priscilla's pulse was thready, bowstring, and rapid overall. In particular, her cubit or most proximal pulse positions corresponding to the kidneys were floating as well.

Taken as a whole, these signs and symptoms added up to liver blood-kidney yin and yang vacuity with vacuity heat disturbing the heart spirit above. Therefore, the treatment principles were to enrich the kidneys and nourish the liver, invigorate yang and clear vacuity heat above. The formula she was given contained the following ingredients:

Rhizoma Curculiginis Orchioidis (*Xian Mao*), 9g
Herba Epimedii (*Xian Ling Pi*), 9g
Radix Angelicae Sinensis (*Dang Gui*), 9g
Rhizoma Anemarrhenae Aspheloidis (*Zhi Mu*), 9g
Cortex Phellodendri (*Huang Bai*), 9g
Fructus Levis Tritici Aestivi (*Fu Xiao Mai*), 45g
Fructus Schisandrae Chinensis (*Wu Wei Zi*), 9g
Concha Ostreae (*Mu Li*), 18g
Herba Ecliptae Prostratae (*Han Lian Cao*), 15g
Fructus Ligustri Lucidi (*Nu Zhen Zi*), 15g

Priscilla took this prescription the same way Gary did above. In addition, she received press needles in the ear acupuncture points *Shen Men* (Spirit Gate), Internal Secretion, Adrenals, and Kidneys, two points in one ear and the other two in the other ear. Priscilla was instructed to press each of these needles four times each day: before bed, after arising, in the morning, and in the afternoon. Further, she was instructed to drink a warm glass of boiled milk in which had been whipped a whole egg.

Within a week, Priscilla reported that her feet were no longer cold and that she no longer was getting up to urinate at night. Since she was not being awoken to pee, she was sleeping six or seven hours each night instead of four. In order to consolidate this treatment, Priscilla received weekly body acupuncture for another six weeks, and she was given the core prescription above as a patent pill. This resulted in her hot flashes and nights sweats going away. In addition, her husband was happy that his wife's libido had returned to its previous level of interest. Since Priscilla's vaginal lubrications also increased (they had been a little dry since menopause), Priscilla found she enjoyed sex a whole lot more.

Carolyn

Carolyn was 32 years old. A year ago she had decided to go back to graduate school. She had been studying hard with considerable mental strain. After all, it is not easy being a single mom, a breadwinner, and a graduate student all at the same time. Hence, Carolyn began to suffer from insomnia. She had great difficulty falling asleep and tossed and turned for hours each night. When she was able to fall asleep, she had nightmares and other very vivid, very disturbing dreams. Often she would wake in a startle, her heart pounding. In school, she noticed that her memory was getting worse, instead of better.

When questioned by her Chinese doctor, Carolyn reported that she also suffered from heart palpitations, restlessness, shortness of breath, and was feeling very withdrawn and uncommunicative. When she was pressed by others into talking, she often became irritable. She was generally fatigued and occasionally had night sweats, especially during her menstruation. Sometimes she had a good appetite, but other times she didn't have the energy to eat. Her bowel movements and urination were both normal and her menstrual cycle was pretty regular. However, since having her little girl two years previously, Carolyn had noticed that the volume of her menses was definitely reduced. For the last year, she had noticed that her insomnia was worse before and during her menses and that she had premenstrual breast distention and discomfort which disappeared as soon as her menses came. On inspection, Carolyn's tongue was red at the tip and had yellow, slimy fur. Her pulse was bowstring, thready, and rapid.

Carolyn's Chinese pattern discrimination was depressive heat disturbing her heart spirit complicated by qi and blood vacuity. The treatment principles were to course the liver and rectify the qi, clear heat and resolve depression, supplement the qi and blood and quiet the spirit. Therefore, Carolyn was given body acupuncture every other day, three days a week at:

Tai Chong (Liv 3)
San Yin Jiao (Sp 6)
Zu San Li (St 36)
Shen Men (Ht 7)
Nei Guan (Per 6)
Shan Zhong (CV 17)
Feng Chi (GB 20)
Si Shen Cong (M-HN-1)

In addition, she was prescribed the following Chinese medicinals to be taken as a water-boiled decoction:

Radix Bupleuri (*Chai Hu*), 9g
Cortex Radicis Moutan (*Dan Pi*), 9g
Fructus Gardeniae Jasminoidis (*Shan Zhi Zi*), 9g
Rhizoma Coptidis Chinensis (*Huang Lian*), 4.5g
Cortex Albizziae Julibrissin (*He Huan Pi*), 9g
Caulis Polygoni Multiflori (*Ye Jiao Teng*), 9g
Rhizoma Atractylodis Macrocephalae (*Bai Zhu*), 9g
Sclerotium Poriae Cocos (*Fu Ling*), 12g
Fructus Tritici Aestivi (*Huai Xiao Mai*), 30g
mix-fried Radix Glycyrrhizae (*Gan Cao*), 9g
Fructus Zizyphi Jujubae (*Da Zao*), 10 pieces
Radix Angelicae Sinensis (*Dang Gui*), 9g
Radix Albus Paeoniae Lactiflorae (*Bai Shao*), 18g

Further, Carolyn was given some Lignum Aquilariae Agallochae (*Chen Xiang*) to burn as incense while she was going to bed at night. After three treatments and four days of taking the above Chinese medicinal formula, Carolyn was able to sleep through the night. However, in order to consolidate the treatment effect, she was told to take *Dan Zhi Xiao Yao Wan* (Moutan & Gardenia Rambling Pills) to continue coursing the liver and clearing heat

144

at the same time as supplementing the qi and blood. She was also advised to come in for two or three acupuncture treatments in the week before her menstruation for two or three cycles, since this was the time her insomnia tended to be at its worst. Carolyn was also advised on a regular exercise program and provided with a deep relaxation tape for daily practice. After three cycles, Carolyn had no more insomnia, her mood was improved, and she had no further premenstrual breast distention or pain. Her concentration at school increased and her grades went up. Six months later, she reconciled with her little girl's father.

Mike

Mike was 54 years old and had been suffering from a one year bout of insomnia. He usually woke between 3-4 AM and then found it difficult to fall back asleep. During the day, Mike felt drowsy and suffered from dizziness when standing up quickly and poor memory. Ever since developing insomnia, his appetite had been off, and, if he did eat a good sized meal, his abdomen would become bloated and he would feel full and uncomfortable. Although Mike felt fatigued, he did not feel restless or agitated. Likewise, he felt no special sensations of warmth or cold. His tongue was enlarged with the marks of the teeth along its edges. The fur was thin and white, but the tongue's color was very noticeably pale. Mike's pulse was quite thready and not very forceful for a man. In addition, Mike had been a strict vegan, eating no animal products for the previous 11 years.

Mike's signs and symptoms add up to heart blood-spleen qi vacuity. Therefore, the treatment principles were to nourish the heart, fortify the spleen, and quiet the spirit. This pattern is usually a very easy type of insomnia to treat. It typically responds well to Chinese herbal medicine. Hence Mike was prescribed:

Radix Astragali Membranacei (*Huang Qi*), 18g
Radix Panacis Ginseng (*Ren Shen*), 6g
Rhizoma Atractylodis Macrocephalae (*Bai Zhu*), 9g
Sclerotium Pararadicis Poriae Cocos (*Fu Shen*), 12g
mix-fried Radix Glycyrrhizae (*Gan Cao*), 9g
Fructus Zizyphi Jujubae (*Da Zao*), 6 pieces
Semen Zizyphi Spinosae (*Suan Zao Ren*), 15g
Semen Biotae Orientalis (*Bai Zi Ren*), 12g
Radix Angelicae Sinensis (*Dang Gui*), 9g
Radix Polygalae Tenuifoliae (*Yuan Zhi*), 9g
Radix Auklandiae Lappae (*Mu Xiang*), 9g

Mike took this formula as a water-boiled decoction for two weeks. He was also convinced to add some beef broth and marrow bone soup to his regular diet as well as an occasional egg. In addition, Mike was instructed how to make Semen Zizyphi Spinosae *(Suan Zao Ren)* and rice, Semen Biotae Orientalis *(Bai Zi Ren)* and rice, and Sclerotium Poriae Cocos *(Fu Ling)* and rice porridge. After two weeks, he was sleeping through the night. His tongue was not so pale and he reported that he had more energy than he had for years. In order to keep Mike moving in the right direction, he was instructed to take *Gui Pi Wan* (Restore the Spleen Pills) for 25 out of every 30 days each month for the next several months. On follow-up one year later, there had been no recurrence. Interestingly, on follow-up, Mike reported that his night vision had markedly improved and now he did not hesitate to drive at night.

Anna

Anna was 87 years old. She had had insomnia for years and years. When she lay down at night to sleep, she couldn't stand having anything lying on her chest, and she could never go to sleep if she did not take some sleeping medication. Anna commonly experienced chest pain, chest oppression, and vexatious heat within her heart. At dawn she would often find herself covered in sweat. Her mind was always busy and her heart frequently skipped beats. Besides a bound, slow and irregular pulse, her pulse was also bowstring, while Anna's tongue was purplish red.

Anna's pattern is a common one in older patients suffering from insomnia. Due to a lifetime of injuries and insults to the system and the declining function of the heart and lungs, the blood tends to become static. This static blood then hinders and impairs the engenderment and transformation of fresh or new blood. This leads to blood and yin vacuity with vacuity heat in the heart disturbing the spirit. Therefore, the treatment principles in Anna's case were to nourish and quicken the blood, course and disinhibit the hundreds of vessels, clear the heart and quiet the spirit. The prescription written for Anna consisted of:

uncooked Radix Rehmanniae (*Sheng Di*), 9g
Radix Angelicae Sinensis (*Dang Gui*), 9g
Radix Rubrus Paeoniae Lactiflorae (*Chi Shao*), 9g
Radix Ligustici Wallichii (*Chuan Xiong*), 6g
Flos Carthami Tinctorii (*Hong Hua*), 9g
Semen Pruni Persicae (*Tao Ren*), 9g
Radix Bupleuri (*Chai Hu*), 4.5g
Radix Platycodi Grandiflori (*Jie Geng*), 4.5g
Fructus Citri Aurantii (*Zhi Ke*), 4.5g
Radix Achyranthis Bidentatae (*Niu Xi*), 6g
Rhizoma Coptidis Chinensis (*Huang Lian*), 1.5g
Succinum (*Hu Po*), 4.5g
Radix Glycyrrhizae (*Gan Cao*), 3g

All the above ingredients except the Succinum (powdered Amber) were decocted in water and administered in three divided doses beginning at lunch. This meant that the last dose was given about a half hour before bed. At this time, Anna used the decocted medicinals to wash down the powdered Succinum. Since neither blood vacuity nor blood stasis respond all that quickly to acupuncture, Anna was not needled. Rather, she was encouraged to A) get a massage once a week and B) take this formula for at least one month before passing judgement. Anna said that she hadn't been able to sleep on her own for years in any case, so she didn't mind waiting a little longer before she could go to sleep on her own.

After one month of taking the above medicinals, Anna was able to go to sleep without Western sedatives three out of every five nights. Anna was also very happy that she was not having so many chest pains or palpitations. Her MD was quite impressed by the changes in Anna's heartbeat when he listened to it at her next checkup. When Anna told him about the Chinese medicinals she had been taking, he said these changes may have only been a "coincidence." However, when Anna was ready to leave, he turned to her and told her that, "If I were you, I'd keep taking those Chinese herbs whatever they are."

As the above case histories show, Chinese medicine treats the whole person. It is not just symptomatic treatment. In all the above cases, the patients not only achieved better sleep but some or all of their other symptoms also "miraculously" disappeared. Actually, there is nothing miraculous about it. If these accompanying symptoms had not disappeared, the Chinese doctor would have thought that that was the funny thing.

Although Chinese medicine does not work immediately the way Western sedatives do, it works without producing drowsiness or a drugged feeling. Even though it usually takes a few days to "kick in", since the whole being feels so much better, it is usually worth the wait and perseverance. In addition, once one understands that Chinese medicine is not a symptomatic "quick fix", this motivates the person to keep on with a good diet, regular exercise, and daily deep relaxation.

Finding a Professional Practitioner of Chinese Medicine

Traditional Chinese medicine is one of the fastest growing holistic health care systems in the West today. At the present time, there are 50 colleges in the United States alone which offer three-four year training programs in acupuncture, moxibustion, Chinese herbal medicine, and Chinese medical massage. In addition, many of the graduates of these programs have done postgraduate studies at colleges and hospitals in China, Taiwan, Hong Kong, and Japan. Further, a growing number of trained Oriental medical practitioners have immigrated from China, Japan, and Korea to practice acupuncture and Chinese herbal medicine in the West.

Traditional Chinese medicine, including acupuncture, is a discreet and independent health care profession. It is not simply a technique that can easily be added to the array of techniques of some other health care profession. The study of Chinese medicine, acupuncture, and Chinese herbs is as rigorous as is the study of allopathic, chiropractic, naturopathic, or homeopathic medicine. Previous training in any one of these other systems does not automatically confer competence or knowledge in Chinese medicine. In order to get the full benefits and safety of Chinese medicine, one should seek out professionally trained and credentialed practitioners.

In the United States, recognition that acupuncture and Chinese medicine are their own independent professions has led to the creation of the National Commission for the Certification of Acupuncture & Oriental Medicine (NCCAOM). This commission has created and administers a national board examination in both acupuncture and Chinese herbal medicine in order to insure minimum levels of professional competence and safety. Those who pass the acupuncture exam append the letters Dipl. Ac. (Diplomate of Acupuncture) after their names, while those who pass the Chinese herbal exam use the letters Dipl. C.H. (Diplomate of Chinese Herbs). I recommend that persons wishing to experience the benefits of acupuncture and Chinese medicine should seek treatment in the U.S. only from those who are NCCAOM certified.

In addition, in the United States, acupuncture is a legal, independent health care profession in more than half the states. A few other states require acupuncturists to work under the supervision of MDs, while in a number of states, acupuncture has yet to receive legal status. In states where acupuncture is licensed and regulated, the names of acupuncture practitioners can be found in the *Yellow Pages* of your local phone book or through contacting your State Department of Health, Board of Medical Examiners, or Department of Regulatory Agencies. In states without licensure, it is doubly important to seek treatment only from NCCAOM diplomates.

When seeking a qualified and knowledgeable practitioner, word of mouth referrals are important. Satisfied patients are the most reliable credential a practitioner can have. It is appropriate to ask the practitioner for references from previous patients treated for the same problem. It is best to work with a practitioner who communicates effectively enough for the patient to feel understood and for the Chinese medical diagnosis and treatment plan to make sense. In all cases, a professional practitioner of Chinese medicine should be able and willing to give a written traditional Chinese diagnosis of the patient's pattern upon request.

For further information regarding the practice of Chinese medicine and acupuncture in the United States of America and for referrals to local professional associations and practitioners in the United States, prospective patients may contact:

National Commission for the Certification of Acupuncture & Oriental Medicine
P.O. Box 97075
Washington DC 20090-7075
Tel: (202) 232-1404
Fax: (202) 462-6157

The National Acupuncture & Oriental Medicine Alliance
14637 Starr Rd, SE
Olalla, WA 98357
Tel: (206) 851-6895
Fax: (206) 728-4841
E mail: 76143.2061@compuserve.com

The American Association of Oriental Medicine
433 Front St.
Catasauqua, PA 18032-2506
Tel: (610) 433-2448
Fax: (610) 433-1832

Learning More About Chinese Medicine

For more information on Chinese medicine in general, see:

The Web That Has No Weaver: Understanding Chinese Medicine by Ted Kaptchuk, Congdon & Weed, NY, 1983. This is the best overall introduction to Chinese medicine for the serious lay reader. It has been a standard since it was first published over a dozen years ago and it has yet to be replaced.

Chinese Secrets of Health & Longevity by Bob Flaws, Sound True, Boulder, CO, 1996. This is a six tape audio cassette course introducing Chinese medicine to laypeople. It covers basic Chinese medical theory, Chinese dietary therapy, Chinese herbal medicine, acupuncture, *qi gong*, *feng shui*, deep relaxation, lifestyle, and more.

Fundamentals of Chinese Medicine by the East Asian Medical Studies Society, Paradigm Publications, Brookline, MA, 1985. This is a more technical introduction and overview of Chinese medicine intended for professional entry level students.

Traditional Medicine in Contemporary China by Nathan Sivin, Center for Chinese Studies, University of Michigan, Ann Arbor, 1987. This book discusses the development of Chinese medicine in China in the last half century.

Imperial Secrets of Health and Longevity by Bob Flaws, Blue Poppy Press, Inc., Boulder, CO, 1994. This book includes a section on Chinese dietary therapy and generally introduces the basic concepts of good health according to Chinese medicine.

Chinese Herbal Remedies by Albert Y. Leung, Universe Books, NY, 1984. This book is about simple Chinese herbal home remedies.

Legendary Chinese Healing Herbs by Henry C. Lu, Sterling Publishing, Inc., NY, 1991. This book is a fun way to begin learning about Chinese herbal medicine. It is full of interesting and entertaining anecdotes about Chinese medicinal herbs.

The Mystery of Longevity by Liu Zheng-cai, Foreign Languages Press, Beijing, 1990. This book is also about general principles and practice promoting good health according to Chinese medicine.

For more information on Chinese dietary therapy, see:

The Dao of Healthy Eating According to Traditional Chinese Medicine by Bob Flaws, Blue Poppy Press, Inc., Boulder, CO, 1997. This book is a layperson's primer on Chinese dietary therapy. It includes detailed sections on the clear, bland diet as well as sections on chronic candidiasis, allergies, and much more.

Prince Wen Hui's Cook: Chinese Dietary Therapy by Bob Flaws & Honora Lee Wolfe, Paradigm Publications, Brookline, MA, 1983. This book is an introduction to Chinese dietary therapy. Although some of the information it contains is dated, it does give the Chinese medicinal descriptions of most foods commonly eaten in the West.

The Book of Jook: Chinese Medicinal Porridges, A Healthy Alternative to the Typical Western Breakfast by Bob Flaws, Blue Poppy Press, Inc., Boulder, CO, 1995. This book is specifically about Chinese medicinal porridges made with very simple combinations of Chinese medicinal herbs.

Chinese Medicinal Wines & Elixirs by Bob Flaws, Blue Poppy Press, Inc., Boulder, CO, 1995. This book is a large collection of simple, one, two, and three Chinese medicinal wines which can be made at home.

Chinese Medicinal Teas: Simple, Proven Folk Formulas for Treating Disease & Promoting Health by Zong Xiao-fan & Gary Liscum, Blue Poppy Press, Inc., Boulder, CO, 1997. Like the above two books, this book is about one, two, and three ingredient Chinese medicinal teas which are easy to make and can be used at home as adjuncts to other, professionally prescribed treatments or for the promotion of health and prevention of disease.

The Tao of Nutrition by Maoshing Ni, Union of Tao and Man, Los Angeles, 1989

Harmony Rules: The Chinese Way of Health Through Food by Gary Butt & Frena Bloomfield, Samuel Weiser, Inc., York Beach, ME, 1985

Chinese System of Food Cures: Prevention & Remedies by Henry C. Lu, Sterling Publishing Co., Inc, NY, 1986

A Practical English-Chinese Library of Traditional Chinese Medicine: Chinese Medicated Diet ed. by Zhang En-qin, Shanghai College of Traditional Chinese Medicine Publishing House, Shanghai, 1990

Eating Your Way to Health — Dietotherapy in Traditional Chinese Medicine by Cai Jing-feng, Foreign Languages Press, Beijing, 1988

Chinese Medical Glossary

Chinese medicine is a system unto itself. Its technical terms are uniquely its own and cannot be reduced to the definitions of Western medicine without destroying the very fabric and logic of Chinese medicine. Ultimately, because Chinese medicine was created in the Chinese language, Chinese medicine is best and really only understood in that language. Nevertheless, as Westerners trying to understand Chinese medicine, we must translate the technical terms of Chinese medicine in English words. If some of these technical translations sound at first peculiar and their meaning is not immediately transparent, this is because no equivalent concepts exist in every-day English.

In the past, some Western authors have erroneously translated technical Chinese medical terms using Western medical or at least quasi-scientific words in an attempt to make this system more acceptable to Western audiences. For instance, the words tonify and sedate are commonly seen in the Western Chinese medical literature even though, in the case of sedate, it meaning is 180° opposite to the Chinese understanding of the word *xie*. *Xie* means to drain off something which has pooled and accumulated. That accumulation is seen as something excess which should not be lingering where it is. Because it is accumulating somewhere where it shouldn't, it is impeding and obstructing whatever should be moving to and through that area. The word sedate comes from the Latin word *sedere*, to sit. Therefore, the word sedate means to make something sit still. In English, we get the word sediment from this same root. However, the Chinese *xie* means draining off something which is sitting somewhere erroneously. Therefore, to think that one is going to sedate what is already sitting is a great mistake in understanding the clinical implication and application of this technical term.

Thus, in order, to preserve the integrity of this system while still making it intelligible to English language readers, I have appended the following glossary of Chinese medical technical terms. The terms themselves are based on Nigel Wiseman's *English-Chinese Chinese-English Dictionary of Chinese Medicine* published by the Hunan Science & Technology Press in Changsha, Hunan, People's Republic of China in 1995. Dr. Wiseman is, I believe, the greatest Western scholar in terms of the translation of Chinese medicine into English. As a Chinese reader myself, although I often find Wiseman's terms awkward sounding at first, I also think they convey most accurately the Chinese understanding and logic of these terms.

Acquired essence: Essence manufactured out of the surplus of qi and blood in turn created out of the refined essence of food and drink

Acupoints: Those places on the channels and network vessels where qi and blood tend to collect in denser concentrations, and thus those places where the qi and blood in the channels are especially available for manipulation

Acupuncture: The regulation of qi flow by the stimulation of certain points located on the channels and network vessels achieved mainly by the insertion of fine needles into these points

Aroma therapy: Using various scents and smells to treat and prevent disease

Ascendant hyperactivity of liver yang: Upwardly out of control counterflow of liver yang due to insufficient yin to hold it down in the lower part of the body

Blood: The red colored fluid which flows in the vessels and nourishes and constructs the tissues of the body

Blood stasis: Also called dead blood, malign blood, and dry blood, blood stasis is blood which is no longer moving through the vessels as it should. Instead it is precipitated in the vessels like silt in a river. Like silt, it then obstructs the free flow of the blood in the vessels and also impedes the production of new or fresh blood.

Blood vacuity: Insufficient blood manifesting in diminished nourishment, construction, and moistening of body tissues

Bowels: The hollow yang organs of Chinese medicine

Channels: The main routes for the distribution of qi and blood, but mainly qi

Clear: The pure or clear part of food and drink ingested which is then turned into qi and blood

Counterflow: An erroneous flow of qi, usually upward but sometimes horizontally as well

Dampness: A pathological accumulation of body fluids

Decoction: A method of administering Chinese medicinals by boiling these medicinals in water, removing the dregs, and drinking the resulting medicinal liquid

Depression: Stagnation and lack of movement, as in liver depression qi stagnation

Drain: To drain off or away some pathological qi or substance from where it is replete or excess

Essence: A stored, very potent form of substance and qi, usually yin when compared to yang qi, but can be transformed into yang qi

Five phase theory: A ancient Chinese system of correspondences dividing up all of reality into five phases of development which then mutually engender and check each other according to definite sequences

Hydrotherapy: Using various baths and water applications to treat and prevent disease

Life gate fire: Another name for kidney yang or kidney fire, seen as the ultimate source of yang qi in the body

Magnet therapy: Applying magnets to acupuncture points to treat and prevent disease

Moxibustion: Burning the herb Artemisia Argyium on, over, or near acupuncture points in order to add yang qi, warm cold, or promote the movement of the qi and blood

Network vessels: Small vessels which form a net-like web insuring the flow of qi and blood to all body tissues

Phlegm: A pathological accumulation of phlegm or mucus congealed from dampness or body fluids

Qi: Activity, function, that which moves, transforms, defends, restrains, and warms

Portals: Also called orifices, the openings of the sensory organs and the opening of the heart through which the spirit makes contact with the world outside

Qi mechanism: The process of transforming yin substance controlled and promoted by the qi, largely synonymous with the process of digestion

Qi vacuity: Insufficient qi manifesting in diminished movement, transformation, and function

Repletion: Excess or fullness, almost always pathological

Seven star hammer: A small hammer with needles embedded in its head used to stimulate acupoints without actually inserting needles

Spirit: The accumulation of qi in the heart which manifests as consciousness, sensory awareness, and mental-emotional function

Stagnation: Non-movement of the qi, lack of free flow, constraint

Supplement: To add to or augment, as in supplementing the qi, blood, yin, or yang

Turbid: The yin, impure, turbid part of food and drink which is sent downward to be excreted as waste

Vacuity: Emptiness or insufficiency, typically of qi, blood, yin, or yang

Vacuity heat: Heat due to hyperactive yang in turn due to insufficient controlling yin

Vessels: The main routes for the distribution of qi and blood, but mainly blood

Viscera: The sold yin organs of Chinese medicine

Yin: In the body, substance and nourishment

Yin vacuity: Insufficient yin substance necessary to both nourish, control, and counterbalance yang activity

Yang: In the body, function, movement, activity, transformation

Yang vacuity: Insufficient warming and transforming function giving rise to symptoms of cold in the body

Index

A

abdominal distention, lower 51, 53, 60

abdominal pain, lower 56, 60

acid regurgitation 55

acupuncture i, 30, 61, 65, 66, 81-84, 86-89, 110, 115, 116, 121, 122, 125, 129-131, 133, 138, 139, 142, 144, 145, 147, 149-151, 153, 158, 160

acupuncture points 30, 61, 82, 88, 115, 121, 122, 133, 142, 160

aerobics 101-103

age & sleep 33

alcohol 4, 43, 46, 83, 92, 95, 99, 100, 122, 123, 129, 140

American Association of Oriental Medicine 151

An Shen Bu Xin Wan 75

antidepressants 4

antihistamines 4

appetite, diminished 51

aroma therapy 114, 115, 128, 158

B

Bai Zi Yang Xin Wan 74

Biotae Nourish the Heart Pills 74

blood 7-13, 17-20, 22, 26, 28, 30, 32-37, 39-43, 45, 47, 51-54, 56-58, 60, 69-77, 79, 81, 82, 85, 87-91, 94-100, 103, 104, 108, 117, 120, 123-127, 135-138, 141, 143, 145, 147, 158-161

Blood Mansion Dispel Stasis Decoction 135

blood stasis 47, 56-58, 69, 79, 87, 135, 137, 147, 159

Bloomfield, Frena 155

Board of Medical Examiners 150

Boulder, CO iii, 111, 153-155

breast distention and pain, premenstrual 51, 60, 64

breast, lumps in the 56

breath, shortness of 54, 84, 143

Bu Nao Wan 74

burping and belching 55

C

Cai Jing-feng 156

causes of insomnia 3, 110

channels & network vessels 28

chest and side of the rib pain 51

China Herb Co. 126

Chinese medicinal porridges 124, 125, 155

Chinese medicinal teas 125, 126, 128, 155

Chinese medicinal wines 123, 124, 155

Chinese Medicinal Wines & Elixirs 155

Chinese patent medicines 68, 69, 80

Chinese self-massage 118, 121, 122, 128

chocolate 92, 94, 99, 140

Cinnabar Sedative Pills 76

Citrus & Pinellia Combination 79

coffee 44, 93, 94, 99, 114, 140

Coptis Warm the Gallbladder Decoction 62, 63

D

Dan Zhi Xiao Yao Wan 71, 79, 144

deep relaxation 89, 104-111, 113, 145, 148, 153

defensive qi 9, 23, 27, 46, 47

Department of Regulatory Agencies 150

depression 2, 3, 17, 41-47, 51-58, 60, 61, 63, 64, 69-72, 74, 75, 78, 79, 82, 84, 85, 87, 90, 93-96, 100, 102-105, 107, 114-117, 119-121, 127, 130, 143, 159

OTHER BOOKS ON CHINESE MEDICINE AVAILABLE FROM:
BLUE POPPY PRESS
5441 Western, Suite 2, Boulder, CO 80301
For ordering 1-800-487-9296 PH. 303\447-8372 FAX 303\245-8362
Email: info@bluepoppy.com Website: www.bluepoppy.com

ACUPOINT POCKET REFERENCE
by Bob Flaws
ISBN 0-936185-93-7
ISBN 978-0-936185-93-4

ACUPUNCTURE & IVF
by Lifang Liang
ISBN 0-891845-24-1
ISBN 978-0-891845-24-6

ACUPUNCTURE AND MOXIBUSTION
FORMULAS & TREATMENTS
by Cheng Dan-an, trans. by Wu Ming
ISBN 0-936185-68-6
ISBN 978-0-936185-68-2

ACUPUNCTURE FOR STROKE REHABILITATION
Three Decades of Information from China
by Hoy Ping Yee Chan, et al.
ISBN 1-891845-35-7
ISBN 978-1-891845-35-2

ACUPUNCTURE PHYSICAL MEDICINE:
An Acupuncture Touchpoint Approach to the
Treatment of Chronic Pain, Fatigue, and Stress
Disorders
by Mark Seem
ISBN 1-891845-13-6
ISBN 978-1-891845-13-0

AGING & BLOOD STASIS:
A New Approach to TCM Geriatrics
by Yan De-xin
ISBN 0-936185-63-6
ISBN 978-0-936185-63-7

A NEW AMERICAN ACUPUNTURE
By Mark Seem
ISBN 0-936185-44-9
ISBN 978-0-936185-44-6

BETTER BREAST HEALTH NATURALLY
with CHINESE MEDICINE
by Honora Lee Wolfe & Bob Flaws
ISBN 0-936185-90-2
ISBN 978-0-936185-90-3

BIOMEDICINE: A Textbook for Practitioners of
Acupuncture and Oriental Medicine
by Bruce H. Robinson, MD
ISBN 1-891845-38-1
ISBN 978-1-891845-38-3

THE BOOK OF JOOK:
Chinese Medicinal Porridges
by B. Flaws
ISBN 0-936185-60-6
ISBN 978-0-936185-60-0

CHANNEL DIVERGENCES
Deeper Pathways of the Web
by Miki Shima and Charles Chase
ISBN 1-891845-15-2
ISBN 978-1-891845-15-4

CHINESE MEDICAL OBSTETRICS
by Bob Flaws
ISBN 1-891845-30-6
ISBN 978-1-891845-30-7

CHINESE MEDICAL PALMISTRY:
Your Health in Your Hand
by Zong Xiao-fan & Gary Liscum
ISBN 0-936185-64-3
ISBN 978-0-936185-64-4

CHINESE MEDICAL PSYCHIATRY
A Textbook and Clinical Manual
by Bob Flaws and James Lake, MD
ISBN 1-845891-17-9
ISBN 978-1-845891-17-8

CHINESE MEDICINAL TEAS: Simple, Proven, Folk
Formulas for Common Diseases & Promoting Health
by Zong Xiao-fan & Gary Liscum
ISBN 0-936185-76-7
ISBN 978-0-936185-76-7

CHINESE MEDICINAL WINES & ELIXIRS
by Bob Flaws
ISBN 0-936185-58-9
ISBN 978-0-936185-58-3

CHINESE MEDICINE & HEALTHY WEIGHT
MANAGEMENT
An Evidence-based Integrated Approach
by Juliette Aiyana, L. Ac.
ISBN 1-891845-44-6
ISBN 978-1-891845-44-4

CHINESE PEDIATRIC MASSAGE THERAPY: A
Parent's & Practitioner's Guide to the Prevention &
Treatment of Childhood Illness
by Fan Ya-li
ISBN 0-936185-54-6
ISBN 978-0-936185-54-5

CHINESE SELF-MASSAGE THERAPY:
The Easy Way to Health
by Fan Ya-li
ISBN 0-936185-74-0
ISBN 978-0-936185-74-3

THE CLASSIC OF DIFFICULTIES:
A Translation of the Nan Jing
translation by Bob Flaws
ISBN 1-891845-07-1
ISBN 978-1-891845-07-9

A COMPENDIUM OF CHINESE MEDICAL
MENSTRUAL DISEASES
by Bob Flaws
ISBN 1-891845-31-4
ISBN 978-1-891845-31-4

CONTROLLING DIABETES NATURALLY WITH
CHINESE MEDICINE
by Lynn Kuchinski
ISBN 0-936185-06-3
ISBN 978-0-936185-06-2

CURING ARTHRITIS NATURALLY WITH
CHINESE MEDICINE
by Douglas Frank & Bob Flaws
ISBN 0-936185-87-2
ISBN 978-0-936185-87-3

CURING DEPRESSION NATURALLY WITH
CHINESE MEDICINE
by Rosa Schnyer & Bob Flaws
ISBN 0-936185-94-5
ISBN 978-0-936185-94-1

CURING FIBROMYALGIA NATURALLY WITH
CHINESE MEDICINE
by Bob Flaws
ISBN 1-891845-09-8
ISBN 978-1-891845-09-3

CURING HAY FEVER NATURALLY WITH
CHINESE MEDICINE
by Bob Flaws
ISBN 0-936185-91-0
ISBN 978-0-936185-91-0

CURING HEADACHES NATURALLY WITH
CHINESE MEDICINE
by Bob Flaws
ISBN 0-936185-95-3
ISBN 978-0-936185-95-8

CURING IBS NATURALLY WITH CHINESE
MEDICINE
by Jane Bean Oberski
ISBN 1-891845-11-X
ISBN 978-1-891845-11-6

CURING INSOMNIA NATURALLY WITH
CHINESE MEDICINE
by Bob Flaws
ISBN 0-936185-86-4
ISBN 978-0-936185-86-6

CURING PMS NATURALLY WITH CHINESE
MEDICINE
by Bob Flaws
ISBN 0-936185-85-6
ISBN 978-0-936185-85-9

DISEASES OF THE KIDNEY & BLADDER
by Hoy Ping Yee Chan, et al.
ISBN 1-891845-37-3
ISBN 978-1-891845-35-6

THE DIVINE FARMER'S MATERIA MEDICA
A Translation of the Shen Nong Ben Cao
translation by Yang Shou-zhong
ISBN 0-936185-96-1
ISBN 978-0-936185-96-5

DUI YAO: THE ART OF COMBINING
CHINESE HERBAL MEDICINALS
by Philippe Sionneau
ISBN 0-936185-81-3
ISBN 978-0-936185-81-1

ENDOMETRIOSIS, INFERTILITY AND
TRADITIONAL CHINESE MEDICINE:
A Laywoman's Guide
by Bob Flaws
ISBN 0-936185-14-7
ISBN 978-0-936185-14-9

THE ESSENCE OF LIU FENG-WU'S
GYNECOLOGY
by Liu Feng-wu, translated by Yang Shou-zhong
ISBN 0-936185-88-0
ISBN 978-0-936185-88-0

EXTRA TREATISES BASED ON INVESTIGATION &
INQUIRY:
A Translation of Zhu Dan-xi's Ge Zhi Yu Lun
translation by Yang Shou-zhong
ISBN 0-936185-53-8
ISBN 978-0-936185-53-8

FIRE IN THE VALLEY: TCM Diagnosis & Treatment
of Vaginal Diseases
by Bob Flaws
ISBN 0-936185-25-2
ISBN 978-0-936185-25-5

FU QING-ZHU'S GYNECOLOGY
trans. by Yang Shou-zhong and Liu Da-wei
ISBN 0-936185-35-X
ISBN 978-0-936185-35-4

FULFILLING THE ESSENCE:
A Handbook of Traditional & Contemporary
Treatments for Female Infertility
by Bob Flaws
ISBN 0-936185-48-1
ISBN 978-0-936185-48-4

GOLDEN NEEDLE WANG LE-TING: A 20th
Century Master's Approach to Acupuncture
by Yu Hui-chan and Han Fu-ru, trans. by Shuai Xue-zhong
ISBN 0-936185-78-3
ISBN 978-0-936185-78-1

A HANDBOOK OF TCM PATTERNS
& THEIR TREATMENTS
by Bob Flaws & Daniel Finney
ISBN 0-936185-70-8
ISBN 978-0-936185-70-5

A HANDBOOK OF TRADITIONAL
CHINESE DERMATOLOGY
by Liang Jian-hui, trans. by Zhang Ting-liang
& Bob Flaws
ISBN 0-936185-46-5
ISBN 978-0-936185-46-0

A HANDBOOK OF TRADITIONAL
CHINESE GYNECOLOGY
by Zhejiang College of TCM, trans. by Zhang Ting-liang
& Bob Flaws
ISBN 0-936185-06-6 (4th edit.)
ISBN 978-0-936185-06-4

A HANDBOOK OF CHINESE HEMATOLOGY
by Simon Becker
ISBN 1-891845-16-0
ISBN 978-1-891845-16-1

A HANDBOOK of TCM PEDIATRICS
by Bob Flaws
ISBN 0-936185-72-4
ISBN 978-0-936185-72-9

THE HEART & ESSENCE OF DAN-XI'S
METHODS OF TREATMENT
by Xu Dan-xi, trans. by Yang Shou-zhong
ISBN 0-926185-50-3
ISBN 978-0-936185-50-7

HERB TOXICITIES & DRUG INTERACTIONS:
A Formula Approach
by Fred Jennes with Bob Flaws
ISBN 1-891845-26-8
ISBN 978-1-891845-26-0

IMPERIAL SECRETS OF HEALTH & LONGEVITY
by Bob Flaws
ISBN 0-936185-51-1
ISBN 978-0-936185-51-4

INSIGHTS OF A SENIOR ACUPUNCTURIST
by Miriam Lee
ISBN 0-936185-33-3
ISBN 978-0-936185-33-0

INTEGRATED PHARMACOLOGY: Combining Modern
Pharmacology with Chinese Medicine
by Dr. Greg Sperber with Bob Flaws
ISBN 1-891845-41-1
ISBN 978-0-936185-41-3

INTRODUCTION TO THE USE OF
PROCESSED CHINESE MEDICINALS
by Philippe Sionneau
ISBN 0-936185-62-7
ISBN 978-0-936185-62-0

KEEPING YOUR CHILD HEALTHY WITH
CHINESE MEDICINE
by Bob Flaws
ISBN 0-936185-71-6
ISBN 978-0-936185-71-2

THE LAKESIDE MASTER'S STUDY OF THE PULSE
by Li Shi-zhen, trans. by Bob Flaws
ISBN 1-891845-01-2
ISBN 978-1-891845-01-7

MANAGING MENOPAUSE NATURALLY WITH
CHINESE MEDICINE
by Honora Lee Wolfe
ISBN 0-936185-98-8
ISBN 978-0-936185-98-9

MASTER HUA'S CLASSIC OF THE
CENTRAL VISCERA
by Hua Tuo, trans. by Yang Shou-zhong
ISBN 0-936185-43-0
ISBN 978-0-936185-43-9

THE MEDICAL I CHING: Oracle of the
Healer Within
by Miki Shima
ISBN 0-936185-38-4
ISBN 978-0-936185-38-5

MENOPAIUSE & CHINESE MEDICINE
by Bob Flaws
ISBN 1-891845-40-3
ISBN 978-1-891845-40-6

TEST PREP WORKBOOK FOR THE NCCAOM BIO-
MEDICINE MODULE: Exam Preparation & Study
Guide
by Zhong Bai-song
ISBN 1-891845-34-9
ISBN 978-1-891845-34-5

POINTS FOR PROFIT: The Essential Guide to
Practice Success for Acupuncturists 3rd Edition
by Honora Wolfe, Eric Strand & Marilyn Allen
ISBN 1-891845-25-X
ISBN 978-1-891845-25-3

PRINCE WEN HUI's COOK: Chinese Dietary Therapy
By Bob Flaws & Honora Wolfe
ISBN 0-912111-05-4
ISBN 978-0-912111-05-6

THE PULSE CLASSIC:
A Translation of the Mai Jing
by Wang Shu-he, trans. by Yang Shou-zhong
ISBN 0-936185-75-9
ISBN 978-0-936185-75-0

THE SECRET OF CHINESE PULSE DIAGNOSIS by
Bob Flaws
ISBN 0-936185-67-8
ISBN 978-0-936185-67-5

SECRET SHAOLIN FORMULAS for the Treatment of
External Injury
by De Chan, trans. by Zhang Ting-liang & Bob Flaws
ISBN 0-936185-08-2
ISBN 978-0-936185-08-8

STATEMENTS OF FACT IN TRADITIONAL
CHINESE MEDICINE   Revise & Expanded
by Bob Flaws
ISBN 0-936185-52-X
ISBN 978-0-936185-52-1

STICKING TO THE POINT 1:
A Rational Methodology for the Step by Step
Formulation & Administration of an Acupuncture
Treatment
by Bob Flaws
ISBN 0-936185-17-1
ISBN 978-0-936185-17-0

STICKING TO THE POINT 2:
A Study of Acupuncture & Moxibustion Formulas
and Strategies
by Bob Flaws
ISBN 0-936185-97-X
ISBN 978-0-936185-97-2

A STUDY OF DAOIST ACUPUNCTURE &
MOXIBUSTION
by Liu Zheng-cai
ISBN 1-891845-08-X
ISBN 978-1-891845-08-6

THE SUCCESSFUL CHINESE HERBALIST
by Bob Flaws and Honora Lee Wolfe
ISBN 1-891845-29-2
ISBN 978-1-891845-29-1

THE SYSTEMATIC CLASSIC OF ACUPUNCTURE
& MOXIBUSTION
A translation of the Jia Yi Jing
by Huang-fu Mi, trans. by Yang Shou-zhong &
Charles Chace
ISBN 0-936185-29-5
ISBN 978-0-936185-29-3

THE TAO OF HEALTHY EATING ACCORDING TO
CHINESE MEDICINE
by Bob Flaws
ISBN 0-936185-92-9
ISBN 978-0-936185-92-7

TEACH YOURSELF TO READ MODERN
MEDICAL CHINESE
by Bob Flaws
ISBN 0-936185-99-6
ISBN 978-0-936185-99-6

TEST PREP WORKBOOK FOR BASIC TCM THEORY
by Zhong Bai-song
ISBN 1-891845-43-8
ISBN 978-1-891845-43-7

TREATING PEDIATRIC BED-WETTING WITH
ACUPUNCTURE & CHINESE MEDICINE
by Robert Helmer
ISBN 1-891845-33-0
ISBN 978-1-891845-33-8

TREATISE on the SPLEEN & STOMACH: A
Translation and annotation of Li Dong-yuan's
Pi Wei Lun
by Bob Flaws
ISBN 0-936185-41-4
ISBN 978-0-936185-41-5

THE TREATMENT OF CARDIOVASCULAR
DISEASES WITH CHINESE MEDICINE
by Simon Becker, Bob Flaws &
Robert Casañas, MD
ISBN 1-891845-27-6
ISBN 978-1-891845-27-7

THE TREATMENT OF DIABETES MELLITUS WITH
CHINESE MEDICINE
by Bob Flaws, Lynn Kuchinski &
Robert Casañas, M.D.
ISBN 1-891845-21-7
ISBN 978-1-891845-21-5

THE TREATMENT OF DISEASE IN TCM, Vol. 1:
Diseases of the Head & Face, Including Mental &
Emotional Disorders
by Philippe Sionneau & Lü Gang
ISBN 0-936185-69-4
ISBN 978-0-936185-69-9

THE TREATMENT OF DISEASE IN TCM, Vol. II:
Diseases of the Eyes, Ears, Nose, & Throat
by Sionneau & Lü
ISBN 0-936185-73-2
ISBN 978-0-936185-73-6

THE TREATMENT OF DISEASE, Vol. III: Diseases
of the Mouth, Lips, Tongue, Teeth & Gums
by Sionneau & Lü
ISBN 0-936185-79-1
ISBN 978-0-936185-79-8

THE TREATMENT OF DISEASE, Vol IV: Diseases of
the Neck, Shoulders, Back, & Limbs
by Philippe Sionneau & Lü Gang
ISBN 0-936185-89-9
ISBN 978-0-936185-89-7

THE TREATMENT OF DISEASE, Vol V: Diseases of
the Chest & Abdomen
by Philippe Sionneau & Lü Gang
ISBN 1-891845-02-0
ISBN 978-1-891845-02-4

THE TREATMENT OF DISEASE, Vol VI: Diseases of
the Urogential System & Proctology
by Philippe Sionneau & Lü Gang
ISBN 1-891845-05-5
ISBN 978-1-891845-05-5

THE TREATMENT OF DISEASE, Vol VII: General
Symptoms
by Philippe Sionneau & Lü Gang
ISBN 1-891845-14-4
ISBN 978-1-891845-14-7

THE TREATMENT OF EXTERNAL DISEASES
WITH ACUPUNCTURE & MOXIBUSTION
by Yan Cui-lan and Zhu Yun-long, trans. by Yang Shou-zhong
ISBN 0-936185-80-5
ISBN 978-0-936185-80-4

THE TREATMENT OF MODERN WESTERN
MEDICAL DISEASES WITH CHINESE MEDICINE
by Bob Flaws & Philippe Sionneau
ISBN 1-891845-20-9
ISBN 978-1-891845-20-8

UNDERSTANDING THE DIFFICULT PATIENT: A
Guide for Practitioners of Oriental Medicine
by Nancy Bilello, RN, L.ac.
ISBN 1-891845-32-2
ISBN 978-1-891845-32-1

YI LIN GAI CUO (Correcting the Errors in the Forest
of Medicine)
by Wang Qing-ren
ISBN 1-891845-39-X
ISBN 978-1-891845-39-0

70 ESSENTIAL CHINESE HERBAL FORMULAS
by Bob Flaws
ISBN 0-936185-59-7
ISBN 978-0-936185-59-0

160 ESSENTIAL CHINESE READY-MADE
MEDICINES
by Bob Flaws
ISBN 1-891945-12-8
ISBN 978-1-891945-12-3

630 QUESTIONS & ANSWERS ABOUT CHINESE
HERBAL MEDICINE:
A Workbook & Study Guide
by Bob Flaws
ISBN 1-891845-04-7
ISBN 978-1-891845-04-8

260 ESSENTIAL CHINESE MEDICINALS
by Bob Flaws
ISBN 1-891845-03-9
ISBN 978-1-891845-03-1

750 QUESTIONS & ANSWERS ABOUT
ACUPUNCTURE
Exam Preparation & Study Guide
by Fred Jennes
ISBN 1-891845-22-5
ISBN 978-1-891845-22-2